TAME THE FLAME

TAME THE FLAME

Anti-Inflammatory Cookbook for Teens

JAMES DAVIS RUKIN

Copyright © 2024 James Davis Rukin

All rights reserved. This book or any portion thereof may not be reproduced or used in any manner whatsoever without the express written permission of the publisher except for the use of brief quotation in a book review.

ISBNs:

Paperback: 9798338596692

Hardcopy: 9798338593844

FOREWORD

As a Registered Dietitian, it has been a privilege to work with many individuals on their journey to better health, but few have shown the determination and passion for transformation like James. When James was 16, he came to me with a diagnosis of Crohn's disease and a typical teen diet laden with fast food. Our first step together was to shift his diet away from ultra-processed foods, refined carbohydrates, and foods high in saturated fat, sodium, and added sugar, and towards a diet rich in whole foods.

James, who already had a love for the kitchen, embraced this change with remarkable enthusiasm. Cooking his own meals became a cornerstone of his health improvement strategy. This practice allowed him to reduce his intake of ultra-processed foods, increase his consumption of whole foods, and maintain full control over the ingredients in his meals.

In addition to managing his Crohn's disease, James was also a dedicated wrestler. This meant he had a secondary goal of ensuring adequate protein intake to support muscle growth and recovery. Throughout our collaboration, I have been continually impressed by James's ability to balance these nutritional needs and adapt popular dishes to meet his health and fitness goals.

I have had the pleasure of reviewing all the recipes in this cookbook with James. Each recipe is thoughtfully crafted to promote wellness and fitness, combining delicious flavors with nutritional balance. This collection of recipes stands as a testament to James's hard work, creativity, and commitment to health.

I hope that this cookbook inspires you as much as James's journey has inspired me. By cooking these meals, you are not only nourishing your body but also taking a proactive step towards better health and well-being.

Sincerely,

Jacqueline Wyman

Registered Dietitian

ACKNOWLEDGMENTS

Creating this cookbook has been a collaborative effort, and I am deeply thankful to everyone who has supported me along the way.

I would like to thank my nutritionist, **Jacqueline Wyman**, whose expertise and passion for healthy eating have been pivotal in the creation of this book. Her guidance and patience have been incredibly helpful.

I also want to express my profound gratitude to **Maria Azka,** my editor, for her attention to detail and insightful feedback. Her help was essential to the creation of this book.

To my family, your unwavering support and encouragement have been the foundation of this project. Thank you for assisting me, tasting food, and always being there when I needed help. Your love and patience have made this possible.

Isis, thank you for always being there for me. You taught me how to cook, and your support has been invaluable.

A special thank you to **Mount Sinai's Kravis Children's Hospital** and all of my doctors for your exceptional care during my sick periods. Your support made my journey to health and wellness much easier.

Thank you all for your support and for making this cookbook a reality.

INTRODUCTION

I hate cookbooks. But wait—don't put this one down just yet! I know, cookbooks often miss the essence of what cooking is really about. Cooking isn't about obsessing over exact measurements; it's about using your senses—your eyes, nose, taste, and touch—to create something extraordinary. We don't want cooking to become as rigid as baking, where one small mistake can turn your dish into a disaster.

So, why write a cookbook if I hate them so much? On September 20th, 2020, I was diagnosed with Crohn's disease.

Crohn's is a chronic inflammatory condition that targets the digestive tract, with certain foods acting as triggers. High sugar, fat, and certain additives can wreak havoc on your gut. If you want to avoid inflammation, just check the ingredients list—if you can't pronounce it, don't eat it.

This diagnosis meant bidding farewell to burgers, pizza, chicken wings, cookies, brownies—basically, everything delicious. Living on salads forever? No thanks! That's why I wrote this cookbook—to reinvent the unhealthy foods we love by removing the inflammatory triggers and making them even tastier.

Every recipe in this book is designed to be delicious, fun, and worth making again. But here's the one rule: don't follow everything in this book to a T. Add more tomatoes, toss in some chili, or maybe skip that diced cow brain (just kidding, it's not in here). Seriously, use these recipes as a starting point, and make them your own.

And most importantly, have fun!

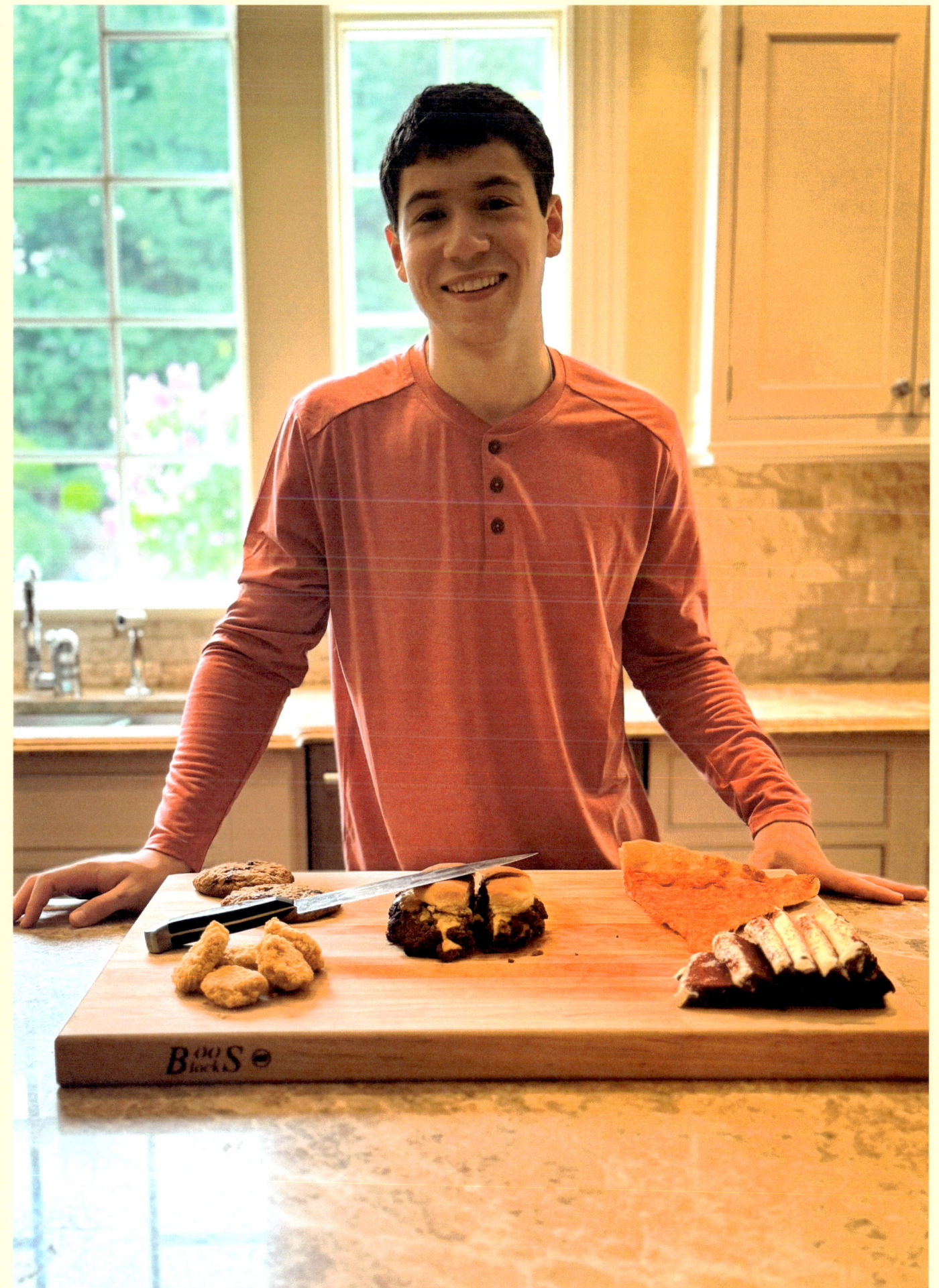

Contents

THE ANTI-INFLAMMATORY FOODS 10
RECIPES
   BASIL PESTO SAUCE 27
   Avocado Crema 29
   Shakshuka 31
   Hummus 33
   Shrimp Tacos 35
   Air-Fried Falafel 37
   Papeta par Eeda 39
   Lemon Tahini Sauce 41
   Tzatziki Sauce 43
   Blueberry & Apple Muffins 45
   Crab Cakes 47
   Grilled Fish Tacos 49
   Spicy Chicken Sandwich 51
   Chicken Sandwich 53
   Light Ranch 55
   Breakfast Sandwich 57
   My Dad's Favorite Breakfast Sandwich 59
   Caesar Salad Dressing 61
   Chicken Caesar Wrap 63
   Chicken Quesadillas 65
   Whole-wheat Tortillas 67
   Mango Fruit Leather 69
   Crustless Quiche 71
   Buffalo Chicken Wings 73
   French Fries 75
   Oatmeal Pancakes 77
   Whole-wheat Pizza Dough 79
   Banana Pancakes 81
   Shrimp Pesto Pizza 83
   Pizza Sauce 85
   How To Stretch Pizza Dough 87

Pappa al Pomodoro	89
Barbecue Sauce	91
Barbecue Chicken Pizza	93
The Best Roasted Chicken	95
Chicken Parmesan	97
Buffalo Ranch Sauce	99
Buffalo Chicken Pizza	101
Chicken Fajitas	103
Chocolate Mousse	105
Flourless Brownie	107
Green Chile Enchiladas	109
Roasted Pepper Pasta	111
The Best Chicken Salad Ever	113
Roasted Tomato Soup	115
Creamy Broccoli Pasta	117
Double Cheeseburger	119
Shrimp Curry	121
Mussels Fra Diavolo	123
Butter Chicken	125
Baingan Bartha	127
Blueberry Glazed Cornbread	129
Lemon and Oregano Octopus	131
Chicken Kebab Wrap	133
Menemen	135
Crunchy Chickpea Snack	137
Birria Tacos	139

THE ANTI-INFLAMMATORY FOODS

LEAFY GREENS

Leafy greens like lettuce, spinach, and kale are rich in antioxidants such as provitamin A carotenoids and vitamin C. They also contain plant compounds like lutein, which is known for its anti-inflammatory properties.

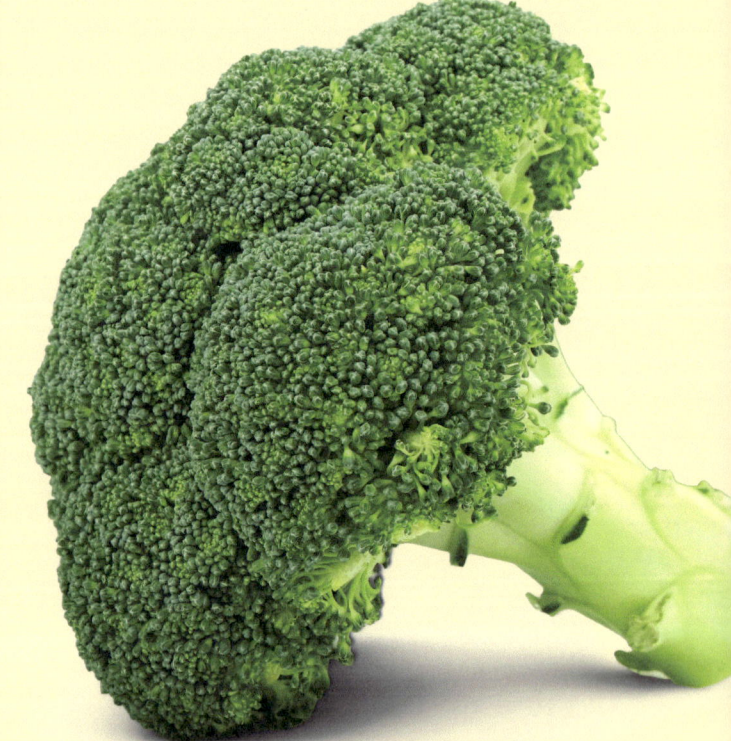

CRUCIFEROUS VEGETABLES

In the family of cruciferous vegetables, we have powerhouses like broccoli, cauliflower, Brussels sprouts, broccoli rabe, radishes, cabbage, kohlrabi, rutabaga, and turnips. This category also embraces nutritious leafy greens such as arugula, bok choy, chard, collard greens, kale, mustard greens, and watercress. These vegetables are renowned not just for their pungent aroma and bold flavors but for their remarkable anti-inflammatory benefits. They are loaded with glucosinolates, which your body converts into isothiocyanates—compounds known to combat inflammation and potentially ward off cancer. Some, like broccoli, Brussels sprouts, and cabbage, are also sources of kaempferol, which is celebrated for its strong anti-inflammatory effects. Moreover, they're a bounty of provitamin A and vitamin C, acting as antioxidants to further reduce inflammation in the body.

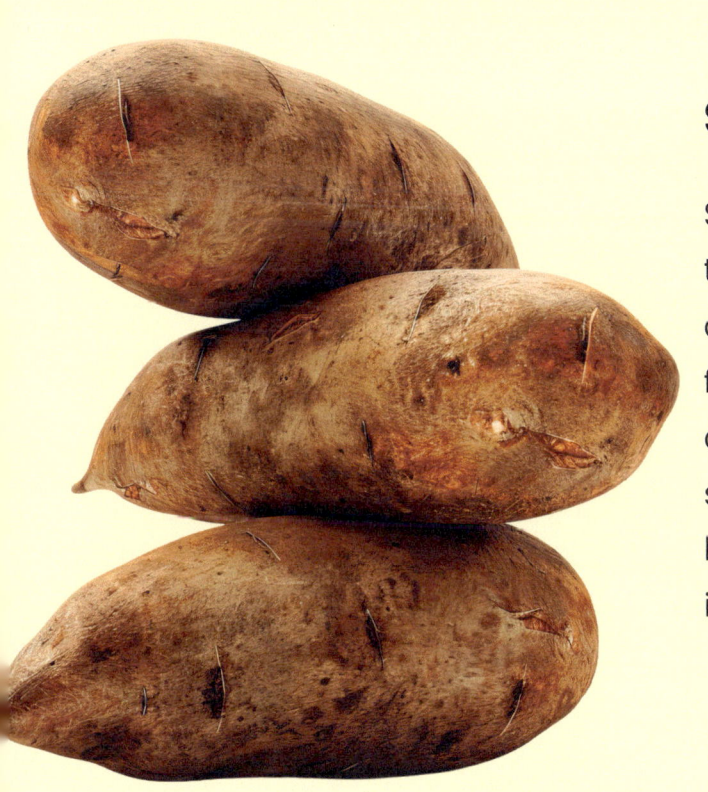

SWEET POTATOES

Sweet potatoes help fight inflammation because they are full of vitamin C, beta-carotene, and antioxidants. These substances reduce harmful free radicals in the body, which can otherwise contribute to inflammation and disease. Purple sweet potatoes are especially good at this because they have anthocyanins, another anti-inflammatory compound.

CARROTS

Carrots contain anti-inflammatory nutrients like beta-carotene, lutein, and polyacetylenes. Different colored carrots have additional compounds like anthocyanins in purple carrots and lycopene in red ones, which may reduce inflammation. Eating carrots in combination with healthy fats can improve the absorption of these beneficial nutrients.

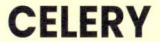

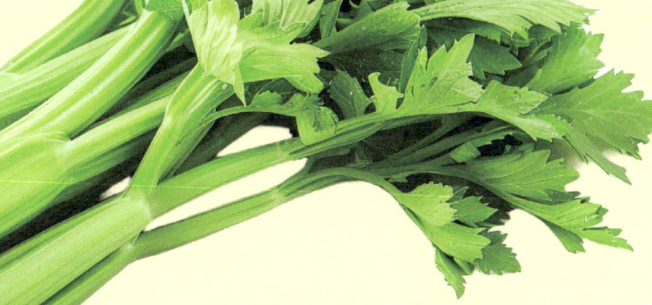

CELERY

Celery's anti-inflammatory potential comes from flavonoids like apigenin. It's mostly water but is still effective at reducing inflammation due to these compounds. It can be eaten in various ways, including in smoothies or as a stuffed snack.

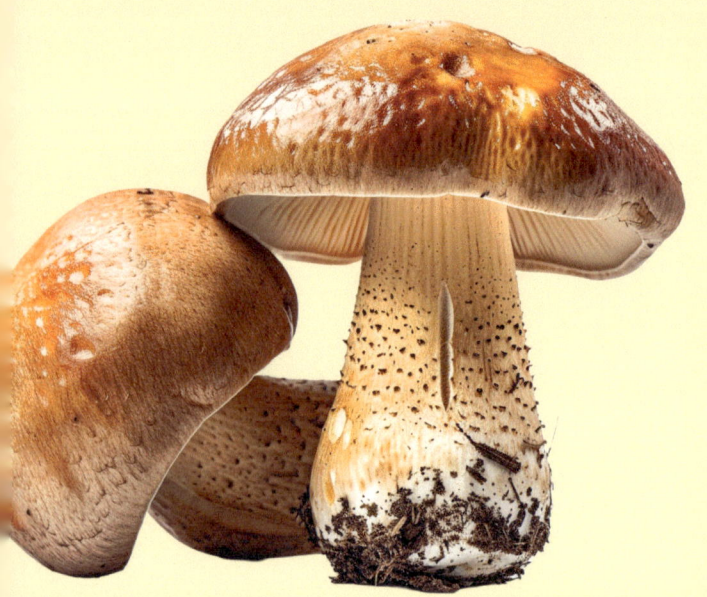

MUSHROOMS

For mushrooms, the key anti-inflammatory agents are polysaccharides, terpenoids, peptides, and phenols. These compounds are different in various mushroom types, with shiitake, porcini, and oyster mushrooms among the varieties offering the greatest benefits. Cooking methods impact their anti-inflammatory potential, with some techniques like steaming or stir-frying preserving more of these helpful substances.

BEETS

Beets contain anti-inflammatory substances known as betalains, which are also antioxidants. The red pigment of beets not only gives them their color but also contains betaine, which may reduce markers of inflammation related to several diseases. Beets are also high in nitrates, which convert to nitric oxide in the body, relaxing blood vessels and offering additional 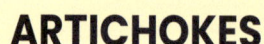 benefits, especially for those with high blood pressure or diabetes.

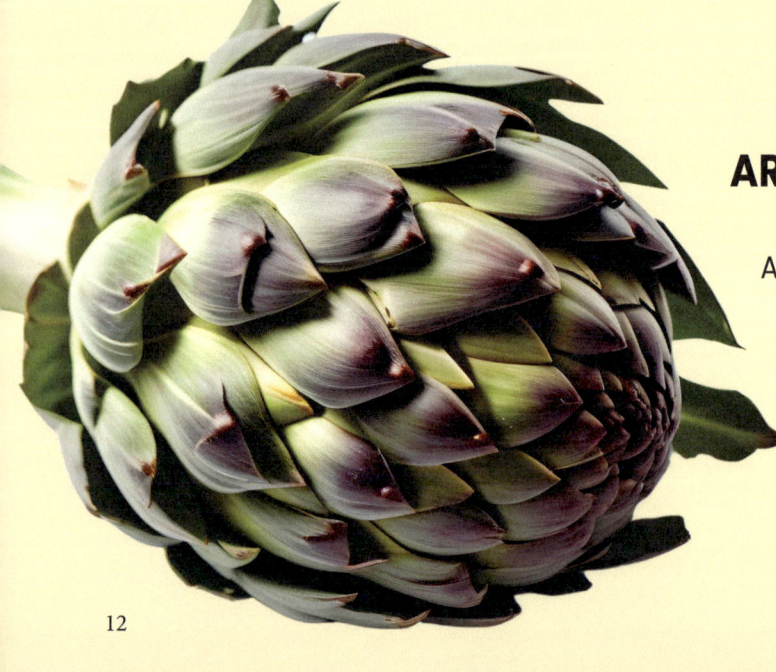

ARTICHOKES

Artichokes are rich in antioxidants and contain anti-inflammatory substances such as cynarin and silymarin. They're also high in fiber, which fosters a healthy gut microbiome, further aiding in reducing inflammation.

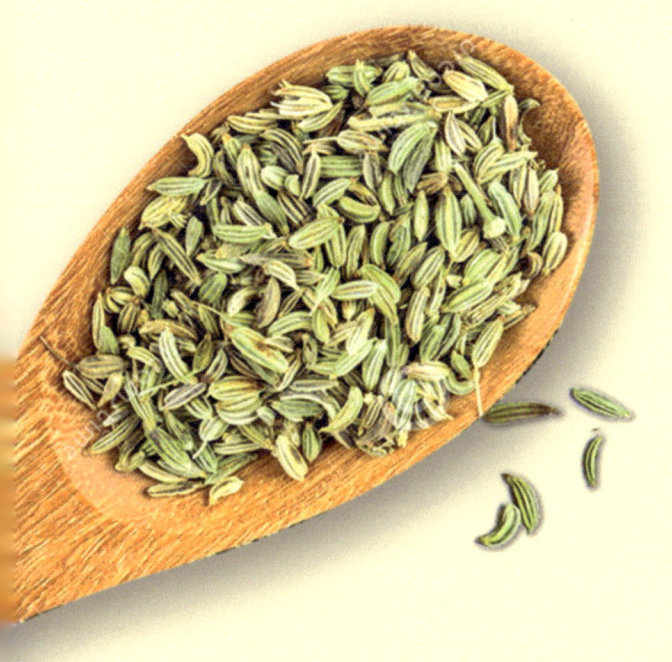

FENNEL

Fennel, with its anise-like flavor, offers anti-inflammatory benefits through compounds like quercetin and anethole. These may ease digestive issues and symptoms of IBD, though conclusive research is ongoing. To maximize benefits, consuming both the bulb and seeds is recommended, and they can be added to broths or salads, or even used to make tea.

CHICORIES

Chicories, such as Belgian endive and radicchio, are full of antioxidants and anti-inflammatory compounds, including anthocyanins that give radicchio its purple color. These nutrients contribute to chicories' anti-inflammatory properties.

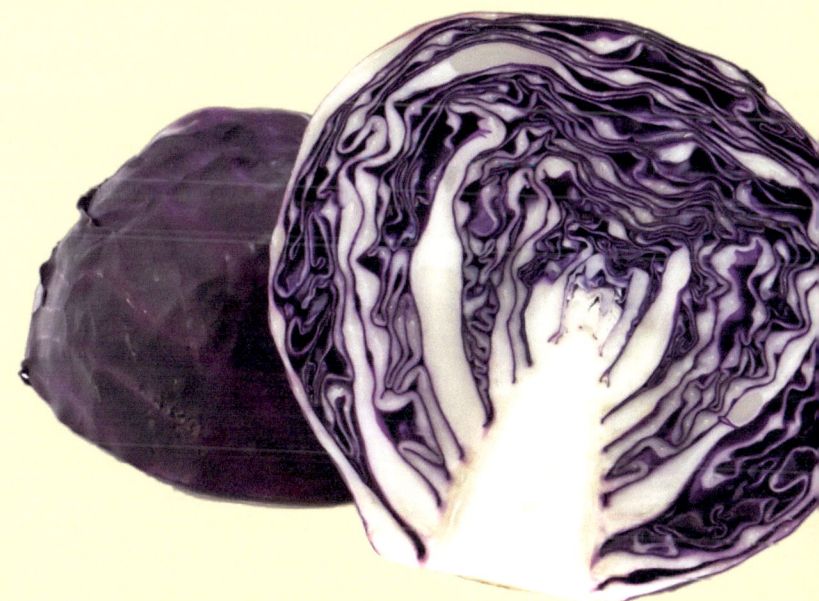

SEA VEGETABLES

Sea vegetables, or seaweeds, are a diverse group providing omega3 fatty acids and antioxidants, which contribute to their anti-inflammatory benefits. They also offer essential amino acids and are good for vegan and vegetarian diets. However, make sure to eat these vegetables in moderation because some of these vegetables contain high levels of iodine, which can cause iodine toxicity.

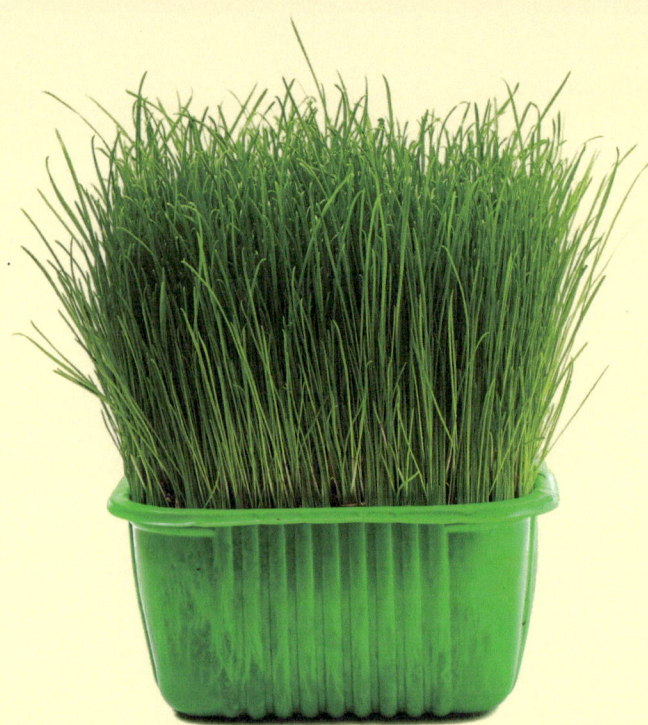

WHEATGRASS

Wheatgrass is lauded for its high chlorophyll content, which has shown potential anti-inflammatory effects. Though not all claims are fully backed by research, wheatgrass may provide benefits in managing inflammation.

PEPPERS

All peppers have anti-inflammatory properties, thanks to vitamin C and capsaicin, with bell peppers being a good source of beta-carotene. However, those with certain medical conditions should be cautious with their pepper intake.

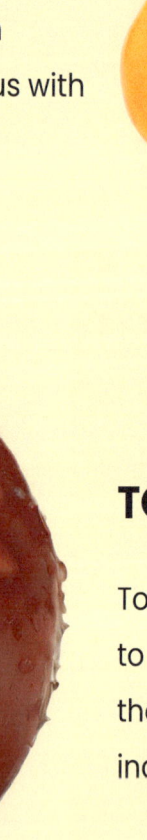

TOMATOES

Tomatoes contain lycopene, an antioxidant linked to reduce inflammation. Cooking tomatoes is thought to enhance the bioavailability of lycopene, increasing their anti-inflammatory potential.

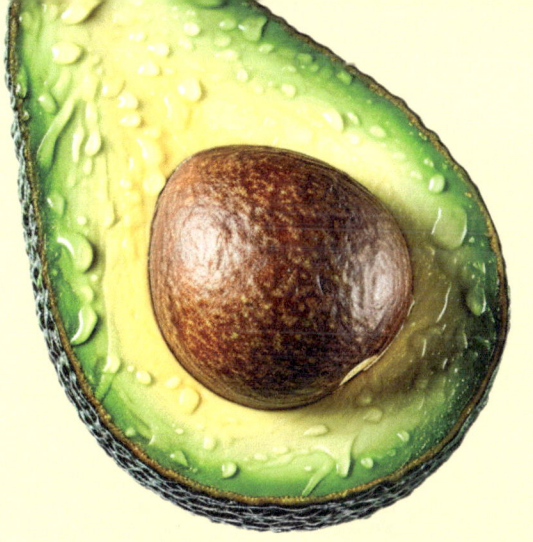

AVOCADOS

Avocados are high in monounsaturated fats and contain carotenoids and other anti-inflammatory nutrients. They're beneficial for heart health and can be incorporated into various meals.

BERRIES

Berries boast high levels of vitamin C, anthocyanins, and other polyphenols, making them powerful agents against inflammation and free radical damage. They support a healthy gut, which is key in managing inflammation.

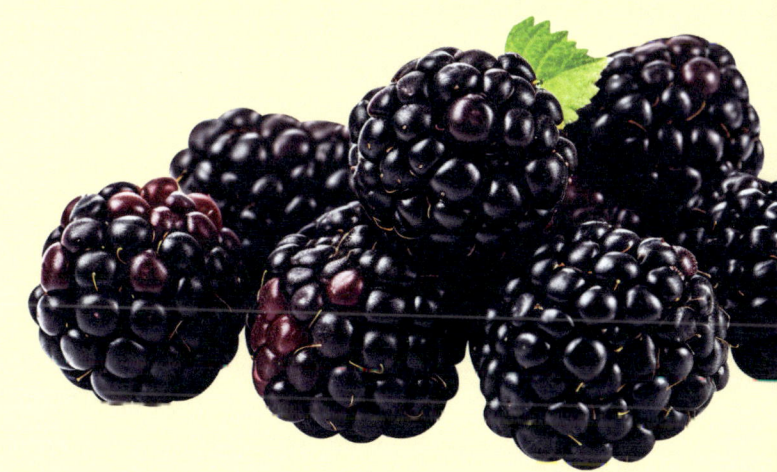

YOGURT

Yogurt's anti-inflammatory effects are attributed to probiotics, which support a robust gut microbiome and optimal immunity. These benefits may extend to a reduction in inflammatory markers. Yogurt can be enjoyed plain or as a component in recipes, and while it's suitable for vegetarian diets that include dairy, there are non-dairy sources of probiotics for those with dairy allergies or lactose intolerance.

CHERRIES

Cherries are rich in antioxidants and polyphenols, which can help reduce inflammation and alleviate symptoms of arthritis. Their high levels of anthocyanins have been shown to decrease inflammatory markers and improve overall joint health.

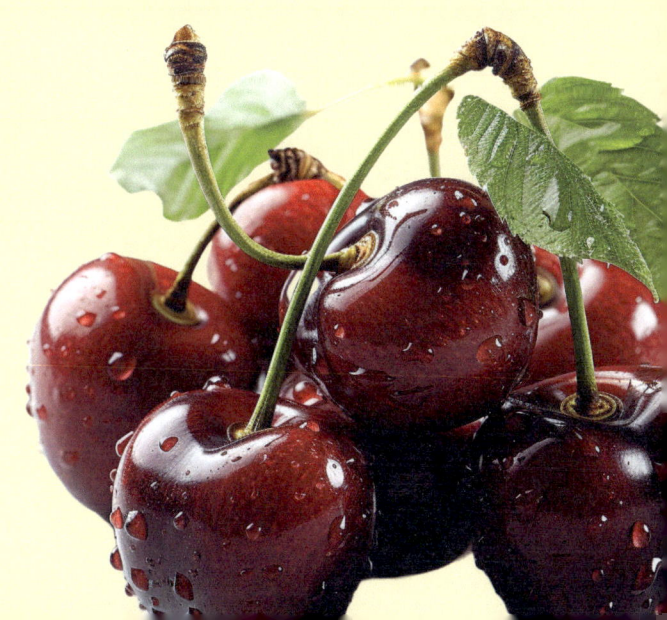

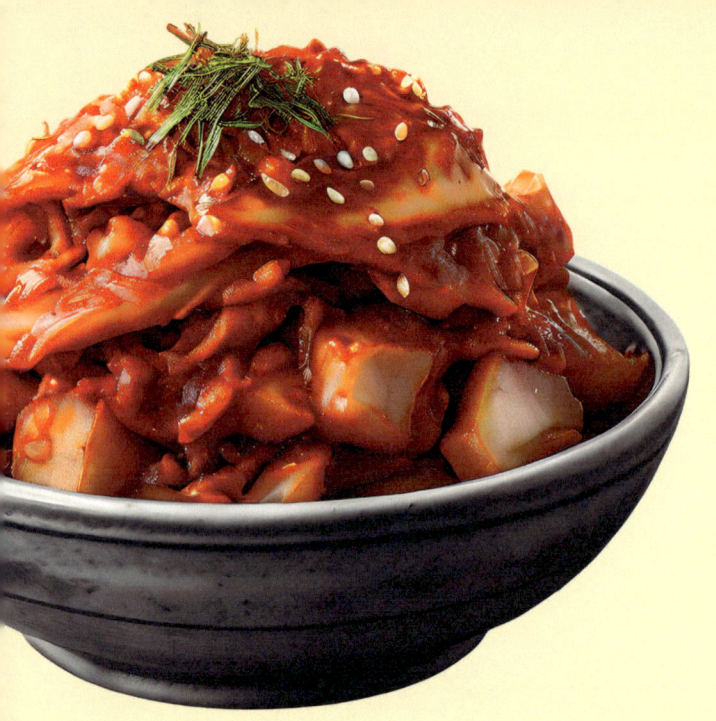

FERMENTED FOODS

Fermented foods like kimchi, sauerkraut, and miso are rich in probiotics due to yeast or bacteria breaking down carbohydrates. These probiotics enhance gut health, bolstering anti-inflammatory processes in the body. It's important to consume them without overheating to maintain live cultures, and they can be incorporated into dressings, bowls, or consumed as a beverage like kombucha.

HONEY

Natural honey contains antioxidants that help manage inflammation and free radicals. It can soothe inflammatory conditions when consumed and even when applied topically. Raw or pure honey is preferred, and it can be used as a natural sweetener or in dressings, although it should be consumed in moderation due to its sugar content.

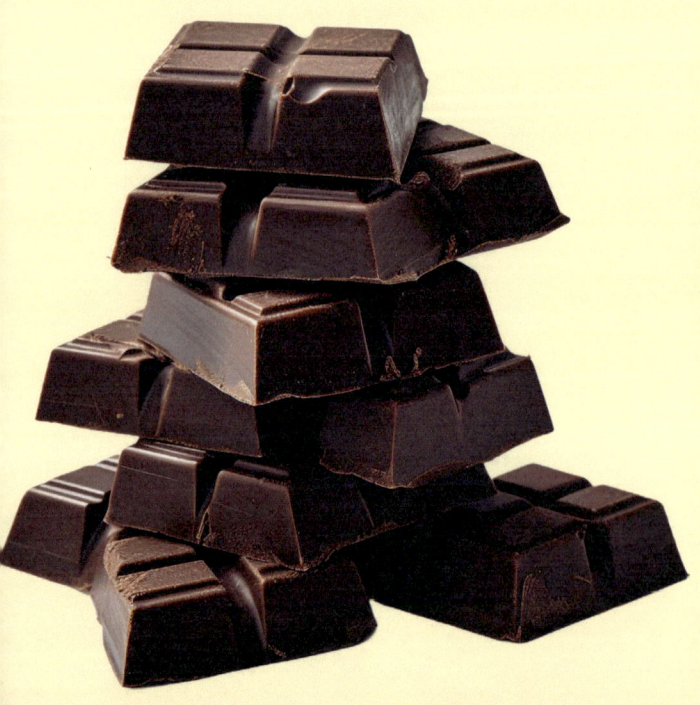

DARK CHOCOLATE

Cocoa in dark chocolate contains flavonoids with antioxidant and anti-inflammatory properties. These may protect against chronic diseases like heart disease. When choosing dark chocolate, opt for high cocoa content and low sugar. It can be consumed on its own or added to recipes, but moderation is key due to its caffeine and oxalate content.

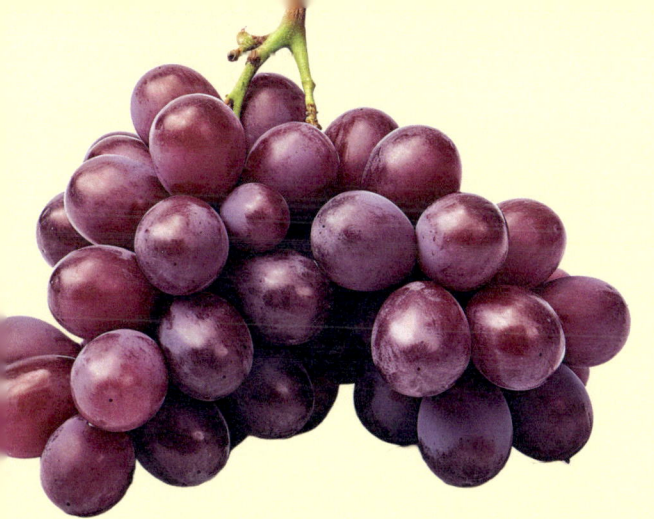

GRAPES

Grapes contain anthocyanins and resveratrol, which protect against damage and inflammation, potentially aiding in disease prevention and longevity.

PINEAPPLE

Pineapple is high in vitamin C and contains bromelain, an enzyme with anti-inflammatory properties that may reduce markers and help with recovery after physical activity.

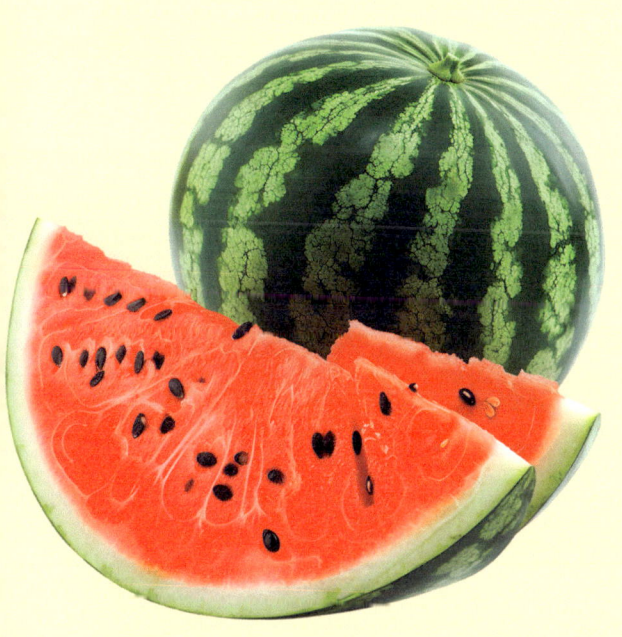

WATERMELON

With lycopene and beta-cryptoxanthin, watermelon may help reduce inflammation and is associated with a decreased risk of rheumatoid arthritis.

CITRUS

Citrus fruits like oranges and grapefruits are loaded with vitamin C, flavonoids, and other compounds that have anti-inflammatory benefits and may help prevent kidney stones.

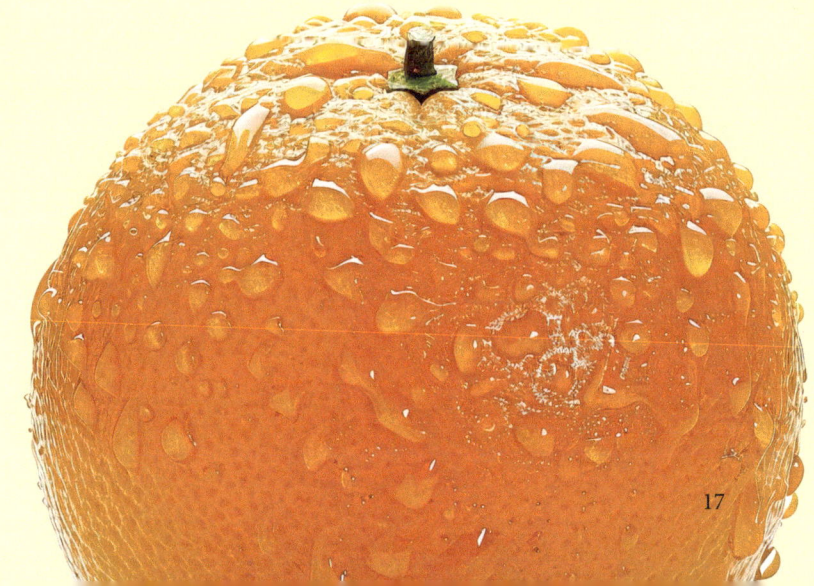

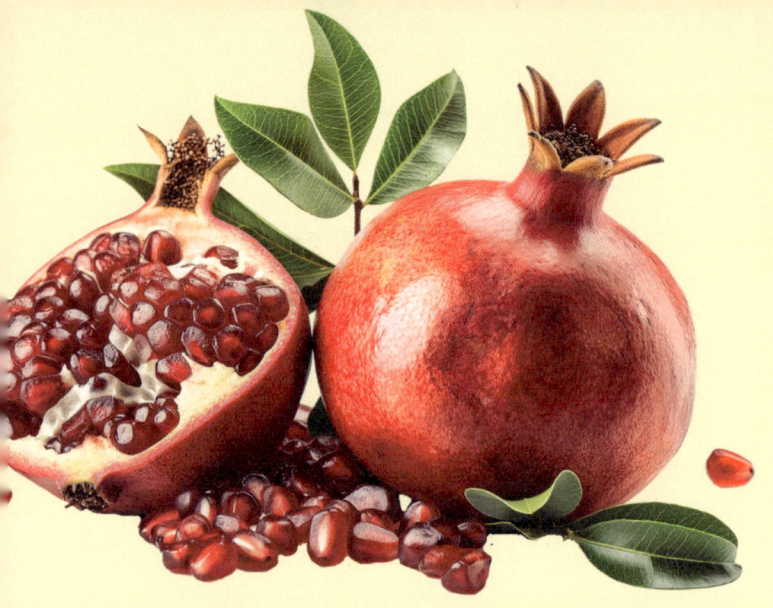

POMEGRANATE

Pomegranates are filled with polyphenols and vitamin C, offering anti-inflammatory benefits that may improve heart health and arthritis symptoms.

CANTALOUPE

Cantaloupe is rich in vitamins A and C and contains the anti-inflammatory carotenoid beta-carotene, which may help lower inflammation in the body.

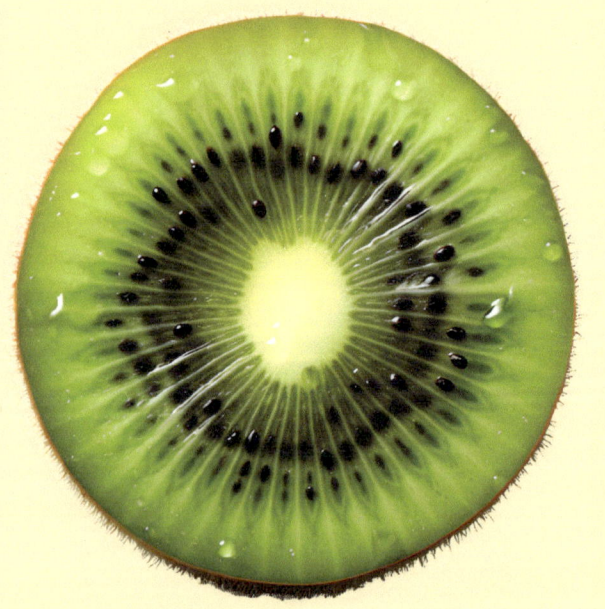

KIWI

Kiwis are antioxidant powerhouses, containing vitamin C and a unique peptide called kissper which may have anti-inflammatory effects. They're especially beneficial for gut health, contributing to a balanced immune response.

APPLE

Apples contain anti-inflammatory polyphenols and fiber. Regular consumption has been associated with reduced levels of inflammatory markers like C-reactive protein, supporting a healthy gut and overall inflammation control.

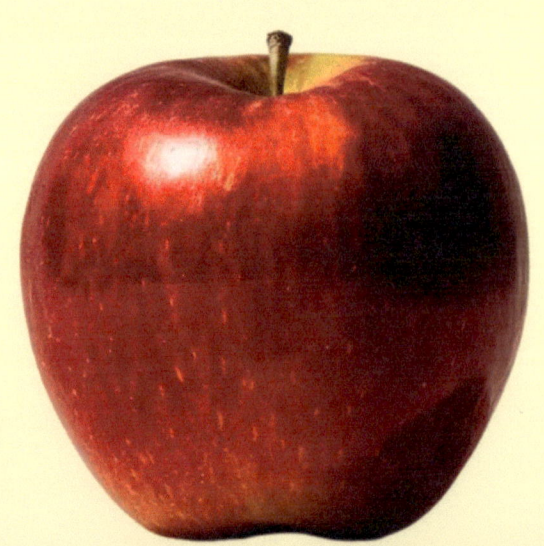

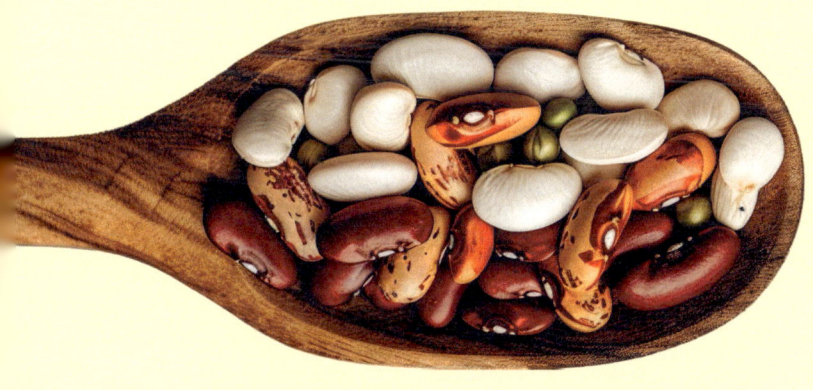

LEGUMES

Beans, peas, and lentils are high in nutrients and antioxidants like polyphenols. They support a healthy gut microbiome due to their fiber content and also provide vitamin C and beta-carotene, enhancing their anti-inflammatory profile.

OATS

Oats are antioxidant-rich, featuring avenanthramides and ferulic acid, which protect against free radicals and may halt the release of pro-inflammatory cytokines. They also offer selenium, supporting antioxidant activity.

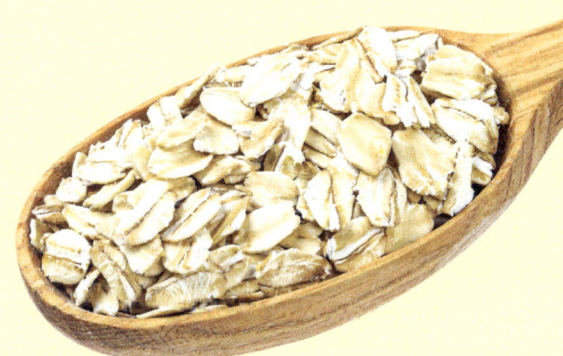

QUINOA

This grain is high in nutrients and anti-inflammatory compounds like fiber and saponins, supporting gut health and reducing inflammation.

RICE

Whole grain rice varieties, particularly brown, black, and red, come packed with inflammation-fighting antioxidants. They have a higher concentration of beneficial compounds like anthocyanins and fiber compared to white rice.

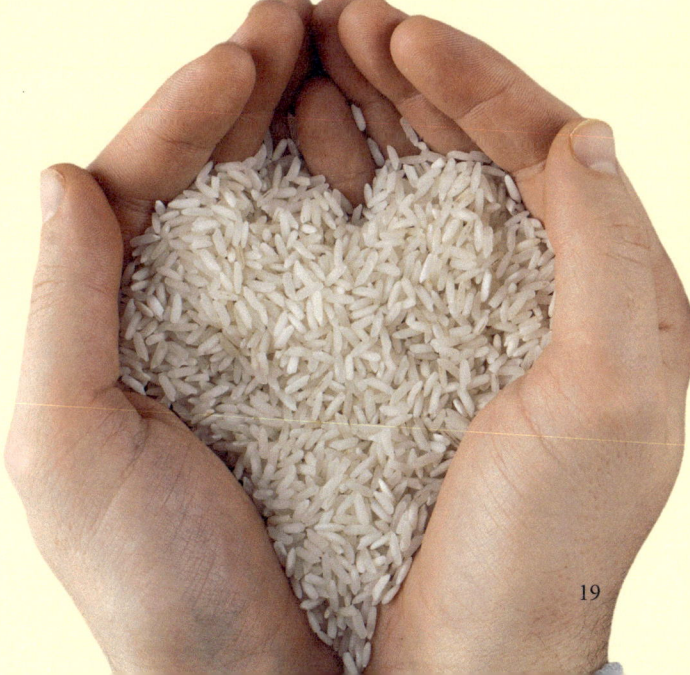

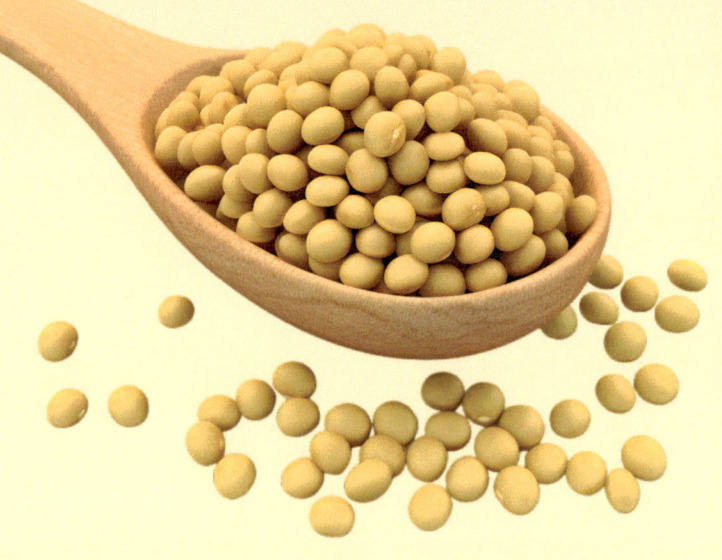

SOYBEANS

Soybeans contain isoflavones and fibers, which have been associated with lowering inflammation and possibly reducing blood levels of C-reactive protein (CRP).

SALMON

Rich in omega-3 fatty acids, salmon is renowned for its anti-inflammatory benefits, helping to decrease the production of inflammation-related compounds in the body.

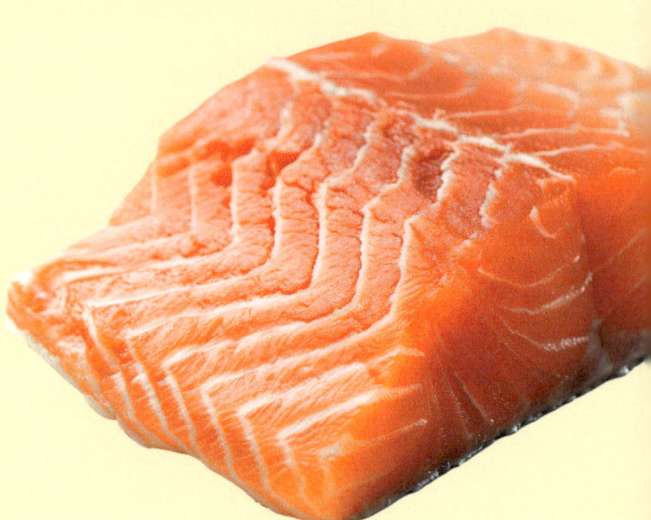

OTHER FATTY FISH/SHELLFISH

Varieties like mackerel and herring offer omega-3 fatty acids, crucial for reducing inflammation and promoting heart health.

WALNUTS

These nuts are packed with anti-inflammatory omega-3 fatty acids and polyphenols, which help combat oxidative stress.

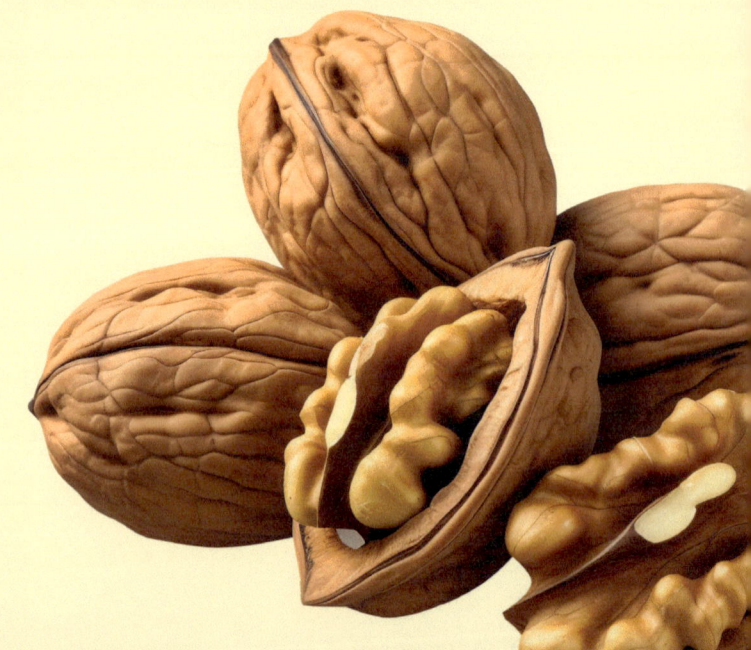

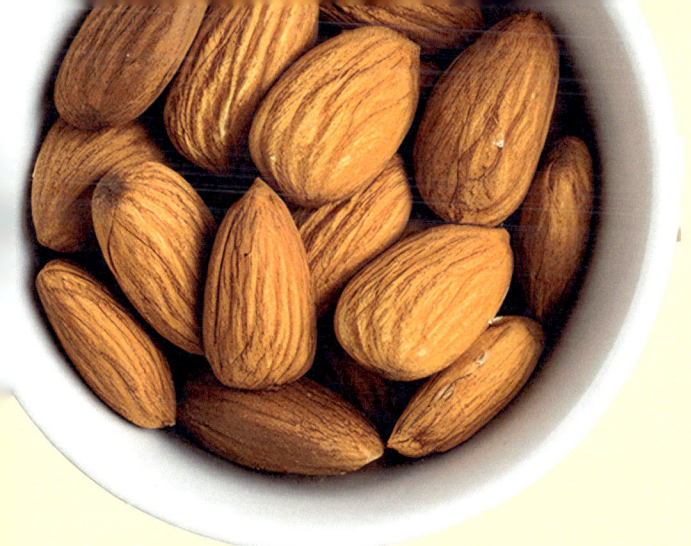

ALMONDS

Almonds are a good source of vitamin E and monounsaturated fats, known for their anti-inflammatory properties.

BRAZIL NUTS

Extremely rich in selenium, Brazil nuts can boost this antioxidant's levels in the body, which is key for preventing cellular damage and inflammation.

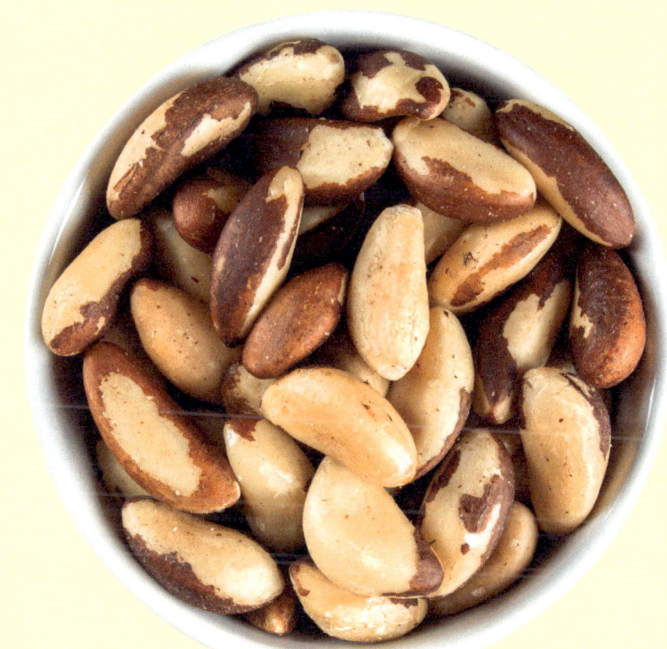

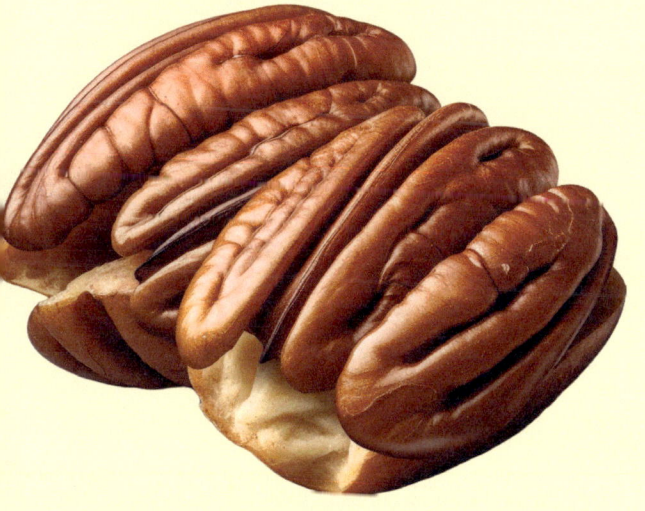

PECANS

Pecans are a good source of monounsaturated fats and dietary fiber. They contain antioxidants such as vitamin E and polyphenols, which can help reduce inflammation and improve heart health. Pecans may also lower bad cholesterol levels (LDL) and could have a protective effect against heart disease.

CHIA SEEDS

Chia seeds are known for their omega-3 fatty acid content, specifically ALA, which can help reduce inflammation. They also contain antioxidants like quercetin and caffeic acid. Chia seeds support a healthy gut due to their fiber content and can be a good addition to a balanced diet to maintain blood sugar levels.

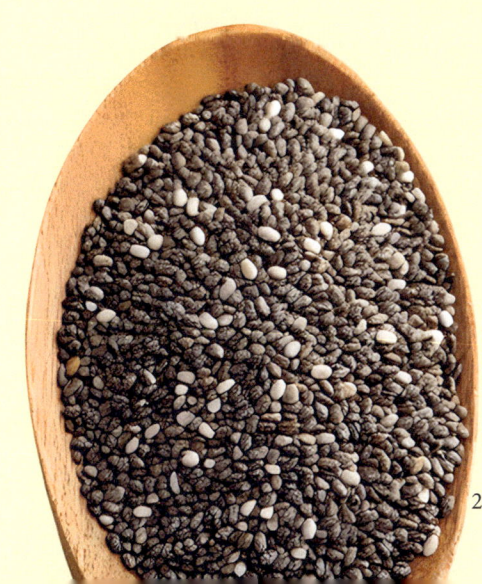

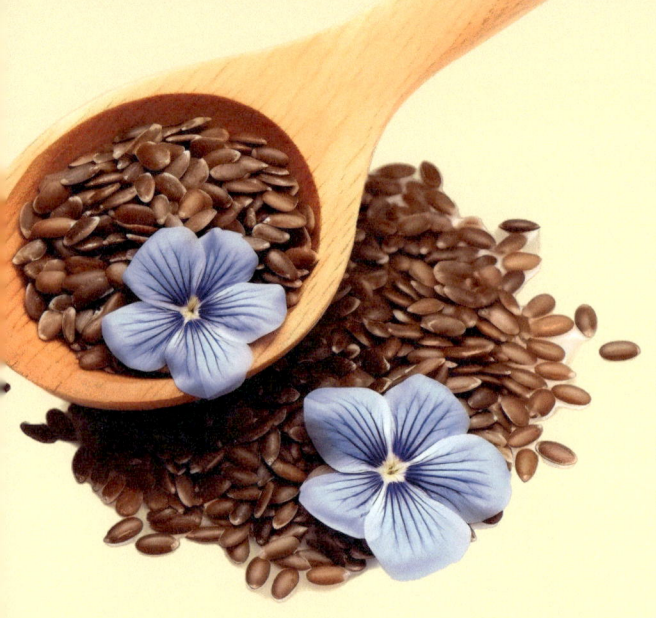

FLAXSEEDS

Flaxseeds are rich in ALA omega-3 fatty acids, which contribute to reducing inflammation. They also contain lignans, a type of phytoestrogen with antioxidant properties, which may help lower inflammation markers and support gut health.

HEMP SEEDS

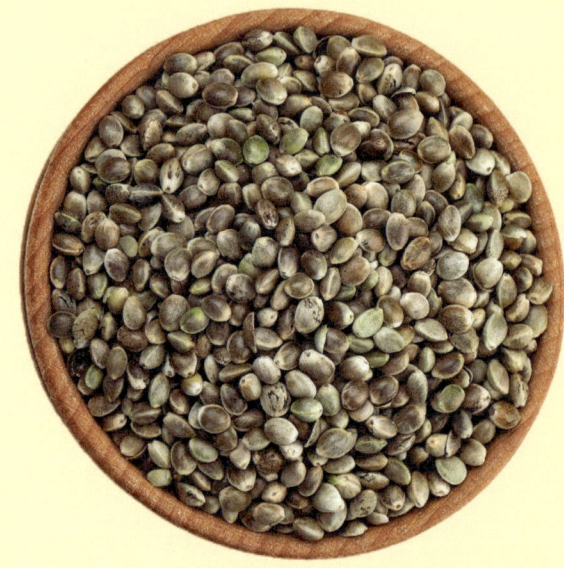

Hemp seeds provide a balanced ratio of omega-3 and omega-6 fatty acids, which are beneficial for reducing inflammation. They are also a good source of plant-based protein and fiber.

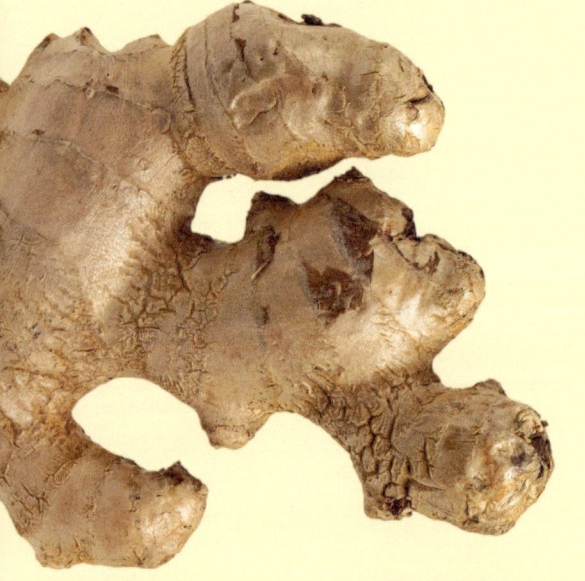

GINGER

Ginger is known for its anti-inflammatory effects and has been used traditionally to alleviate nausea, aid digestion, and relieve pain. It contains gingerol, which has anti-inflammatory and antioxidant properties.

PARSLEY

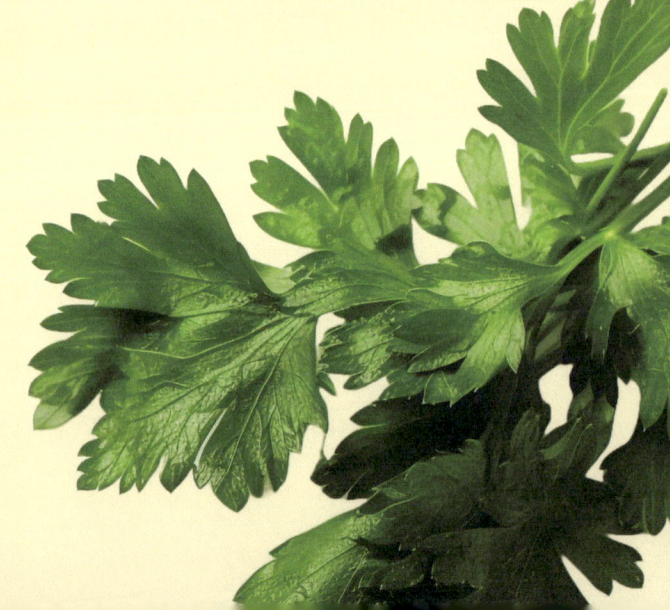

Rich in vitamin C and flavonoids like apigenin, parsley has anti-inflammatory benefits and is also known for its high antioxidant content.

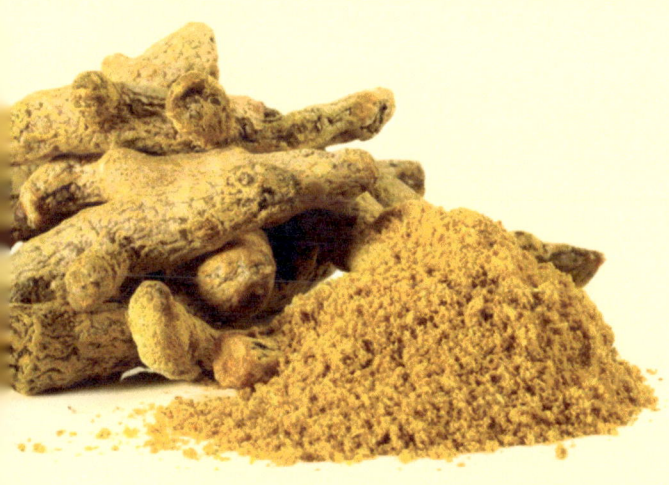

TURMERIC

The active ingredient in turmeric is curcumin, which has potent anti-inflammatory and antioxidant effects. It's been studied for its potential to improve symptoms of arthritis and exercise-induced soreness, among other conditions.

GARLIC

Garlic contains compounds that can help fight inflammation and provide cardiovascular benefits. It has been shown to suppress cytokine production and boost immune health.

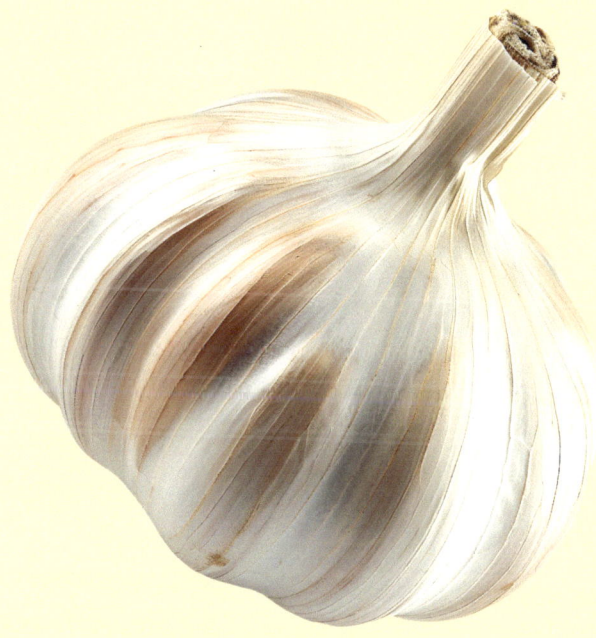

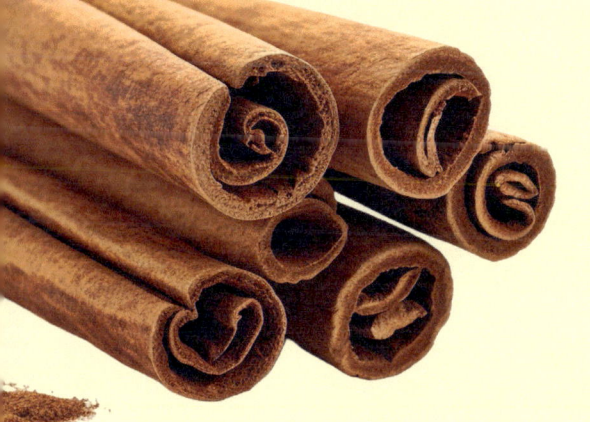

CINNAMON

Cinnamon boasts high levels of antioxidants and has anti-inflammatory properties, potentially helping with blood sugar control and heart health.

GREEN TEA

Green tea is rich in epigallocatechin-3-gallate (EGCG), a catechin with anti-inflammatory properties, which may be protective against various diseases driven by inflammation.

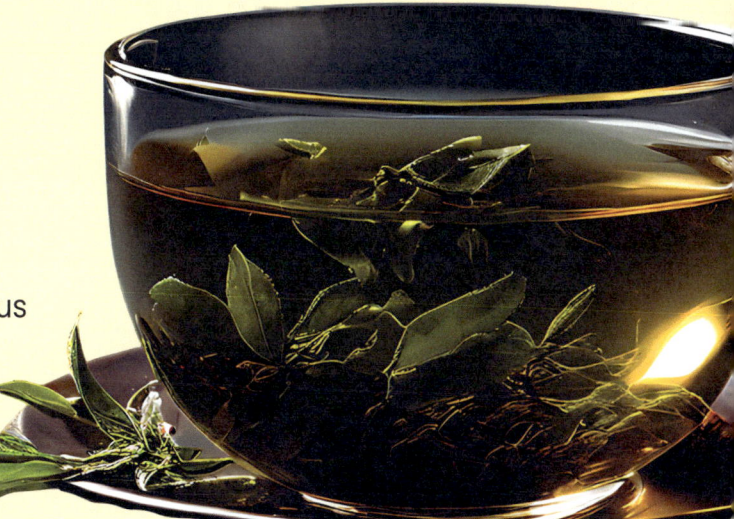

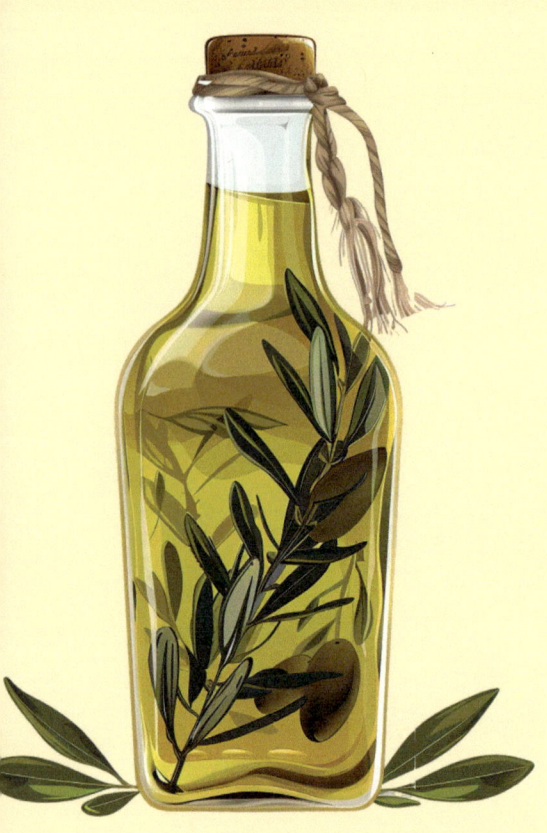

OLIVE OIL

Olive oil is lauded for its content of oleocanthal, an anti-inflammatory compound. It also contains monounsaturated fats, mainly oleic acid, which may reduce inflammation and is associated with heart health benefits.

RECIPES

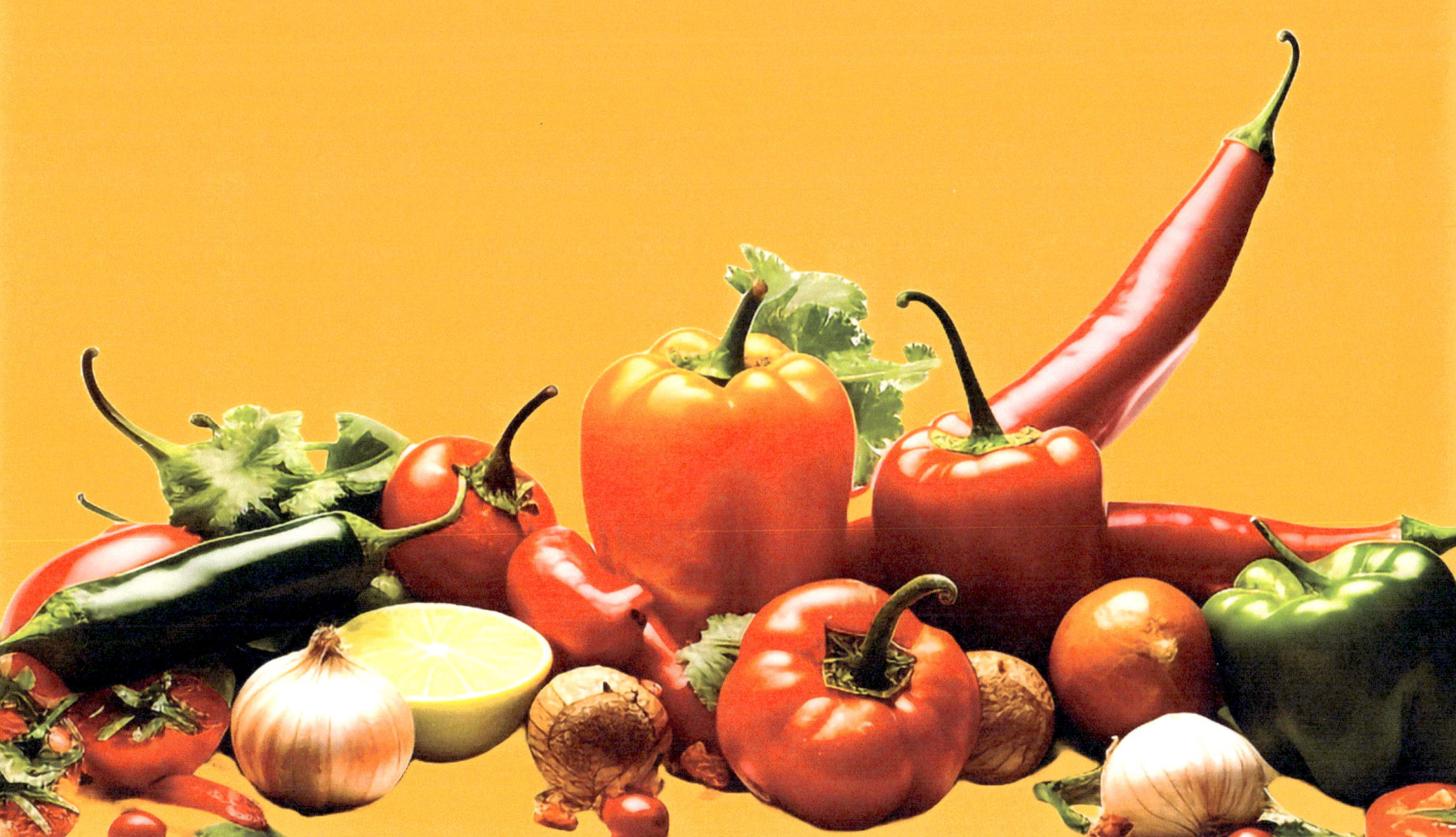

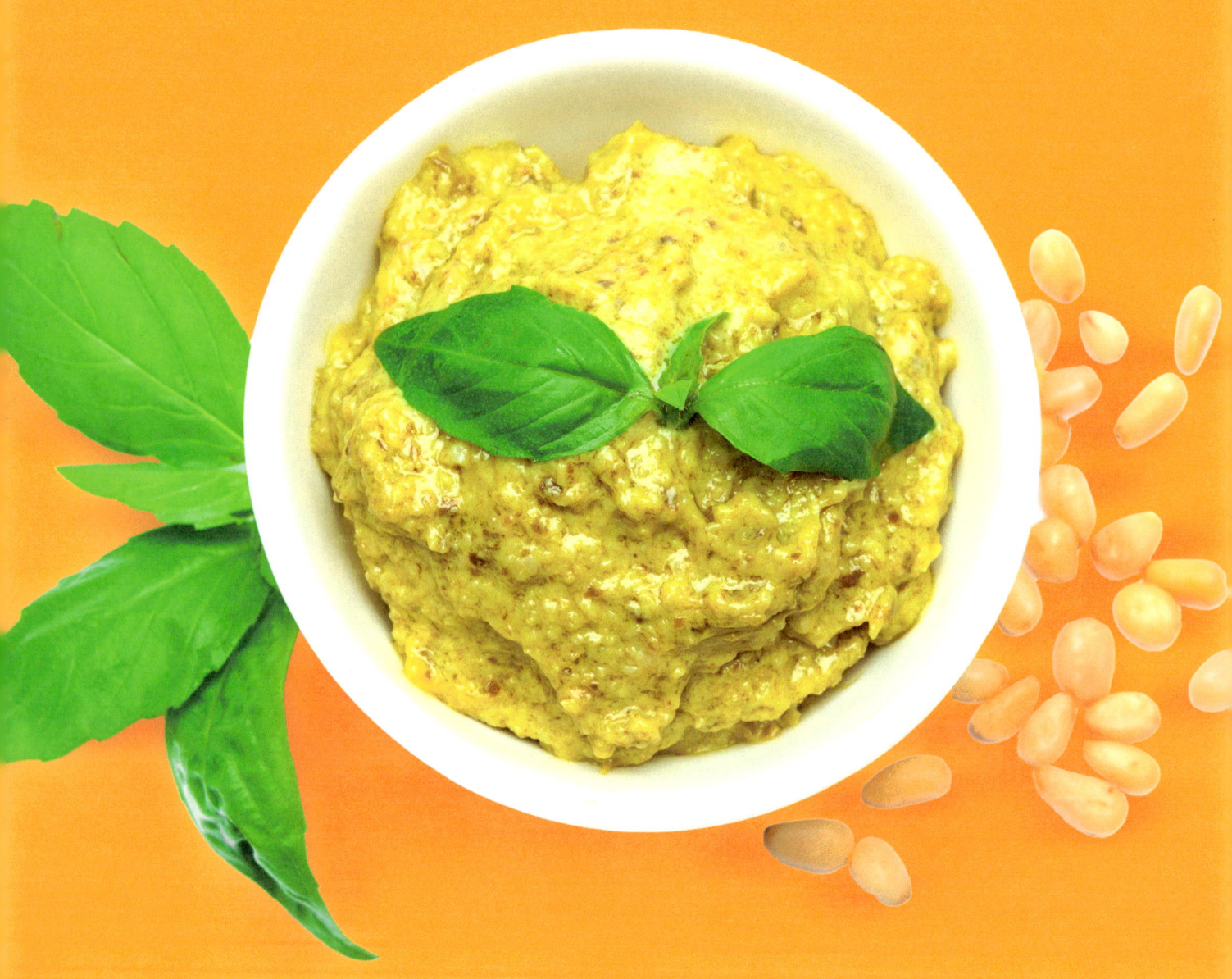

BASIL PESTO SAUCE

BASIL PESTO SAUCE

Fresh, zesty basil pesto that's perfect for pasta or spreading on sandwiches. Seriously, it's a game-changer!

INGREDIENTS

1 bunch (about 1.5 cups) basil leaves

½ cup pine nuts

¼ cup freshly grated Parmesan cheese

2 garllc cloves

¼ C Olive oil

Salt and pepper

METHOD

1. Heat a pan over medium heat. Cook the pine nuts for 2 minutes, stirring constantly until golden brown. Set aside.

2. Preheat the oven to 350°F (175°C).

3. Halve the garlic cloves and place them in a ramekin with olive oil, salt, and pepper. Roast for 15-20 minutes and let cool for 20 minutes.

4. In a food processor, combine basil, pine nuts, roasted garlic with oil, and Parmesan.

5. Blend while gradually adding olive oil until smooth.

6. Season with salt and pepper to taste.

7. Refrigerate until ready to use.

8. Enjoy!

Total Servings	4
Per Serving	
Calories	264.5
Added sugars	0g
Fiber	1.2g
Fat	27.1g
Saturated Fat	4.2g

Values are approximate and may vary based on ingredients used

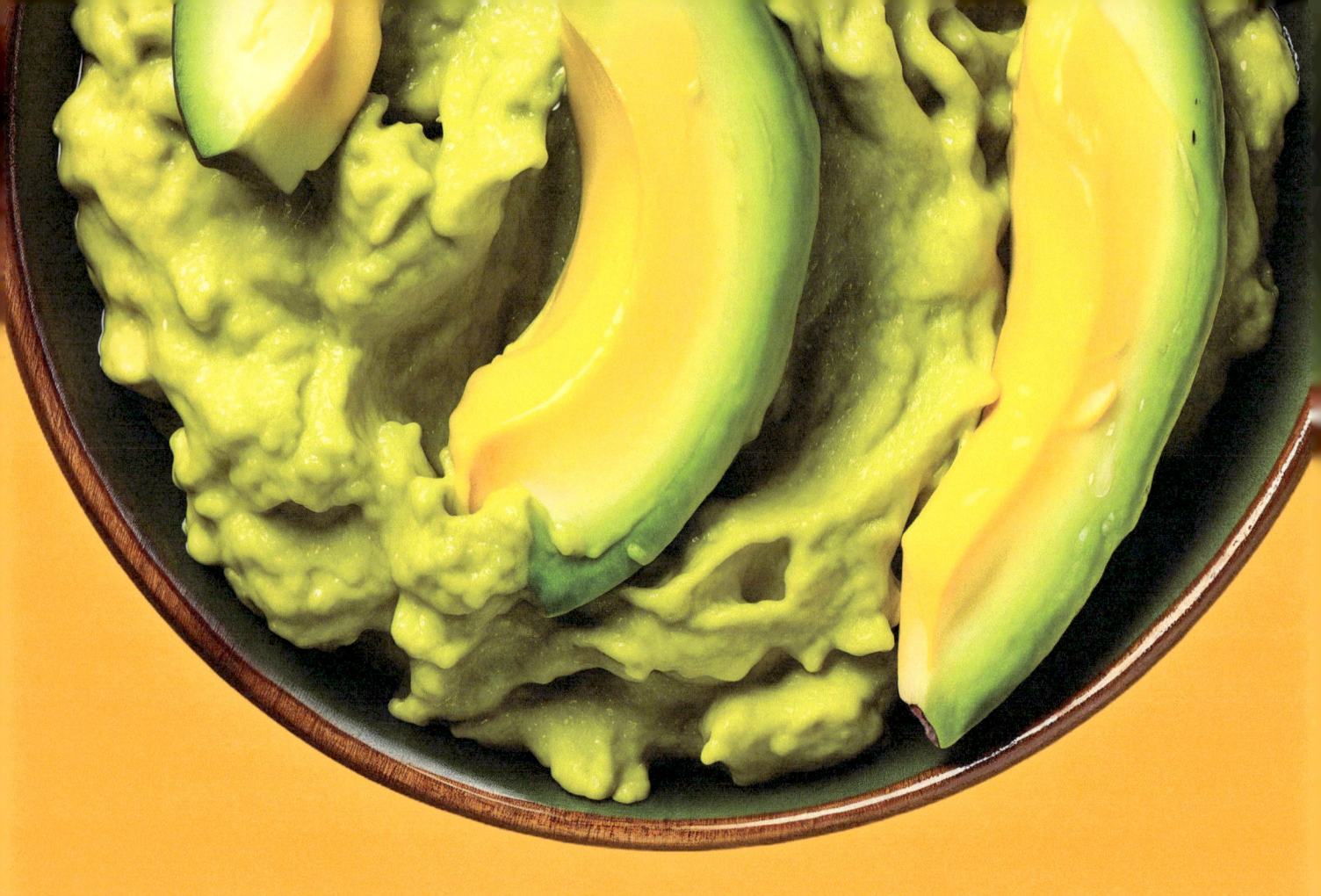

AVOCADO CREMA

AVOCADO CREMA

This creamy, spicy avocado dip is perfect for tacos, burritos, or just dunking your chips in. Yum!

INGREDIENTS

1 avocado

2 tablespoons olive oil

½ jalapeño

½ cup cilantro

1 clove garlic

½ cup lime juice

1 teaspoon diced red onion

Pinch of salt

Pinch of pepper

METHOD

1. Combine all ingredients in a blender.
2. Blend until smooth.
3. Adjust seasoning with salt and pepper as needed.
4. Enjoy!

Total Servings	4
Per Serving	
Calories	123.6
Added Sugar	0g
Fiber	2.6g
Fat	12g
Saturated Fat	1.78g
Protein	0.85g

Values are estimated and can change according to ingredients used

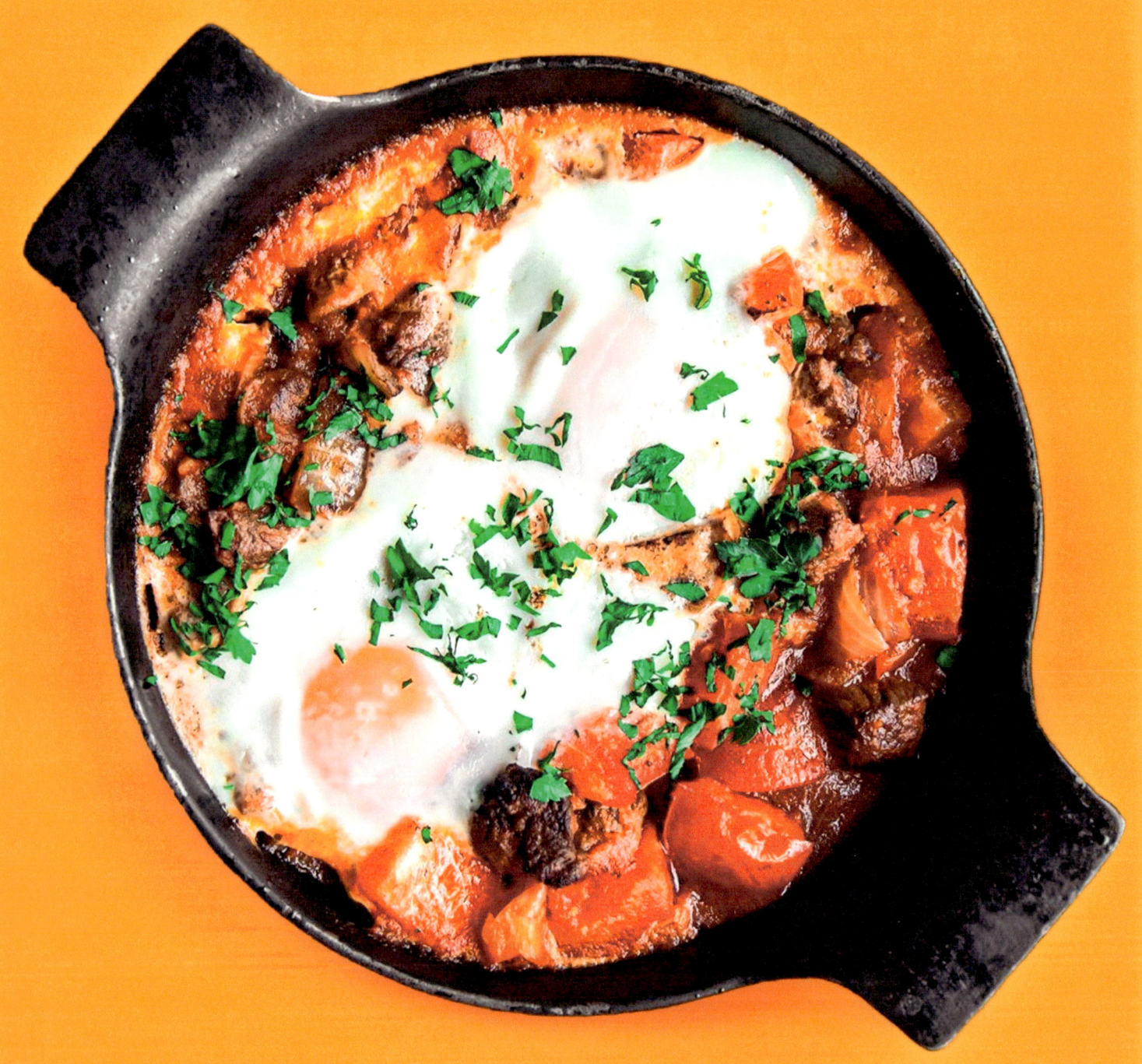

SHAKSHUKA

SHAKSHUKA

Brighten up your breakfast with shakshuka—spicy tomato sauce with poached eggs. It's a flavor explosion

INGREDIENTS

2 tablespoons olive oil

1 medium yellow onion, diced

1 red bell pepper, seeded and diced

4 garlic cloves, finely chopped

2 teaspoons paprika

1 teaspoon cumin

½ teaspoon chili powder

½ teaspoon ground coriander

1 (28-ounce) can whole peeled tomatoes

5 large eggs

Salt and pepper, to taste

¼ cup fresh cilantro, chopped

¼ cup fresh parsley, chopped

½ cup crumbled feta cheese (optional)

1 avocado (optional)

METHOD

1. Heat the olive oil in a medium-sized saucepan over medium heat.

2. Sauté the diced onion and red bell pepper for 5-6 minutes, or until the onion is translucent.

3. Add the garlic, paprika, cumin, chili powder, and ground coriander. Cook for 2 minutes over medium-low heat.

4. Add the entire can of whole peeled tomatoes with juice. Reduce heat to low and mash the tomatoes with a large spoon.

5. Cook the mixture on low for 15-20 minutes until it thickens. The mixture should be thick enough that a spoon leaves a trail when run through it. Season with salt and pepper to taste

6. Make 5 wells in the tomato sauce and crack one egg into each well.

7. Cover the saucepan with a lid and cook for about 7 minutes, or until the eggs are set.

8. Slice the avocado (if using) and lay the slices on a plate.

9. Serve a portion of shakshuka over the avocado slices.

10. Sprinkle with crumbled feta cheese (if using) and garnish with fresh cilantro and parsley.

11. Enjoy!

Total Servings	5
Per Serving	
Calories	174
Added Sugar	0g
Fiber	3.5g
Fat	10.9g
Saturated Fat	2.32g
Protein	8.24g

Values are estimated and not including optional Avocado or Feta

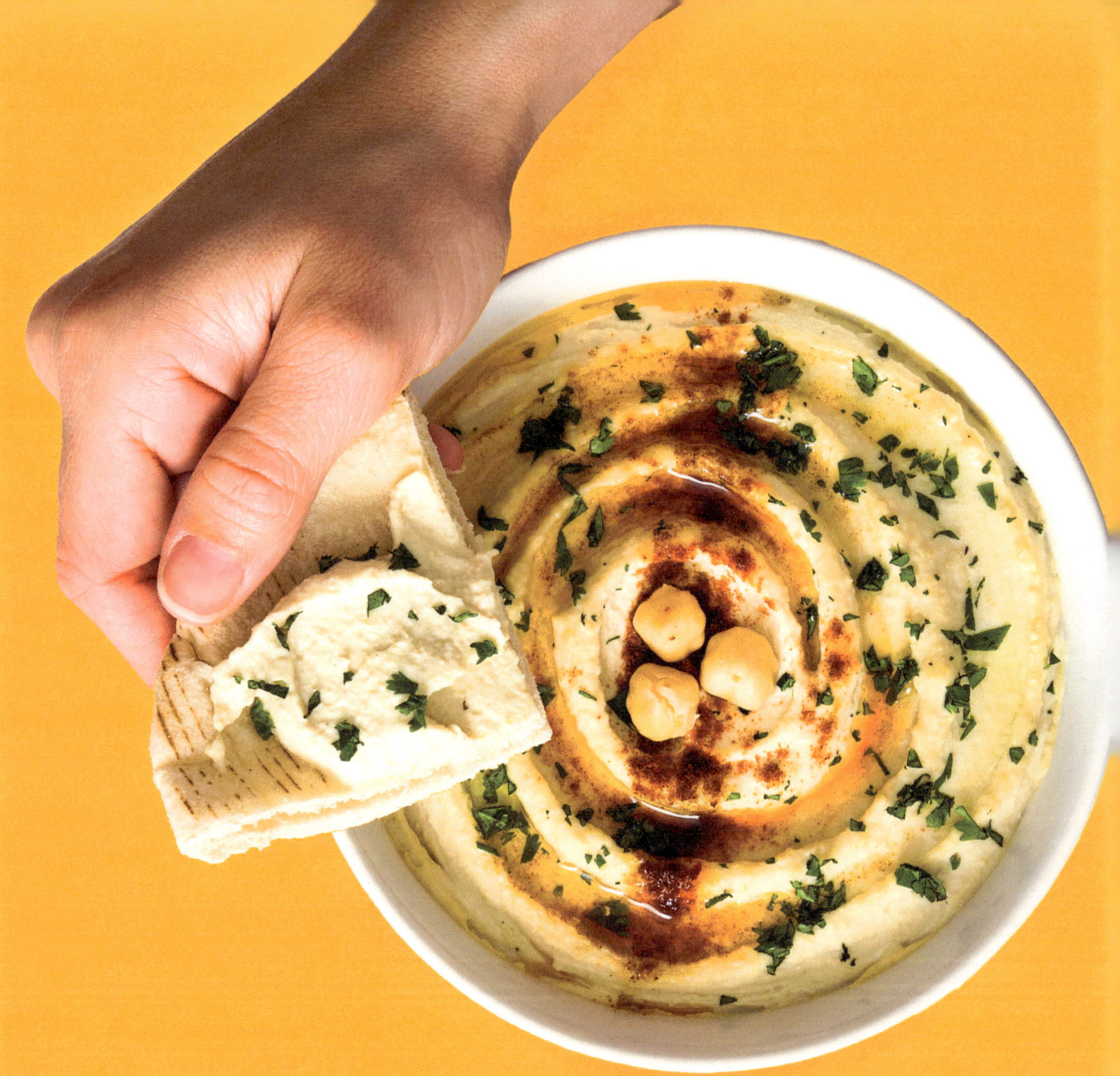

HUMMUS

HUMMUS

Smooth, garlicky hummus that's perfect for dipping veggies or slathering on pita. It's like the best snack ever.

INGREDIENTS

15.5 oz can of chickpeas

½ cup tahini

1 lemon

Ice water

2 garlic cloves

About 2.5 tablespoons olive oil

¾ teaspoon salt

Cumin

METHOD

1. Drain the chickpeas and place them in a bowl of water. Gently massage the chickpeas to remove their skins. Discard the skins. Drain the chickpeas.

2. In a food processor, combine the chickpeas, tahini, juice from the lemon, garlic, and salt.

3. Turn on the food processor and slowly add the olive oil. Adjust the amount based on preference.

4. Every 20 seconds, add a bit of ice water to the food processor.

5. Pulse for 5 minutes, then taste and adjust the seasoning.

6. Pulse for another 5 minutes, taste again, and plate the hummus.

7. Lightly season the surface of the hummus with cumin.

8. Enjoy!

Total Servings	8
Per Serving	
Calories	177.3
Added sugar	0g
Fiber	2.8g
Fat	13.2g
Saturated Fat	1.9g
Protein	5g

Values are approximate and may vary based on ingredients used

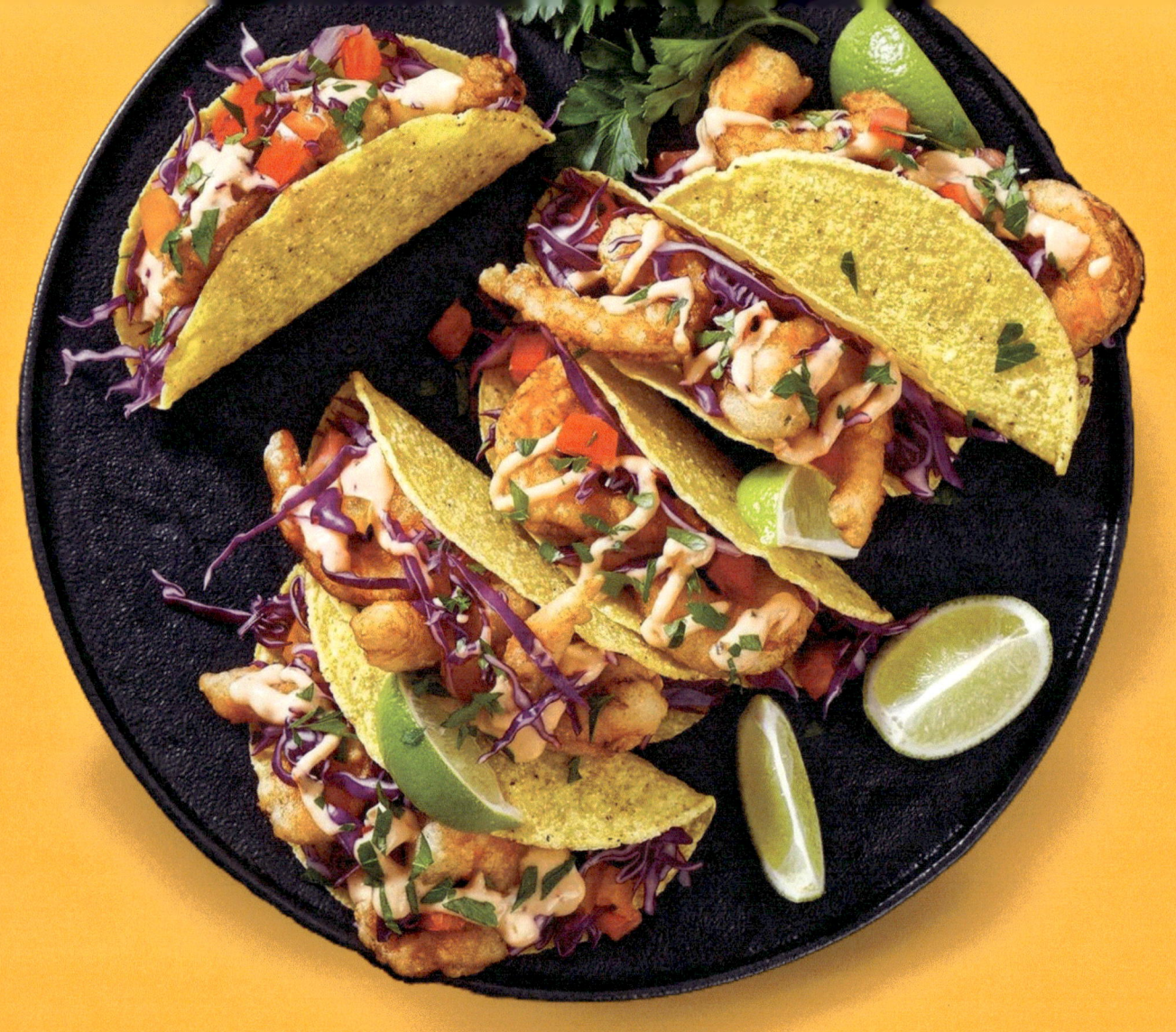

SHRIMP TACOS

SHRIMP TACOS

These shrimp tacos are packed with flavor and perfect for a quick, tasty dinner. Beach vibes, anyone?

INGREDIENTS

FOR THE SHRIMP

40 medium raw shrimp
½ teaspoon cumin
½ teaspoon black pepper
½ teaspoon curry powder
½ teaspoon turmeric
¼ teaspoon ground coriander
½ teaspoon garlic powder
½ teaspoon paprika
2 teaspoons salt
1 tablespoon olive oil

FOR THE CILANTRO LIME SAUCE

Juice of 2 limes
2 cloves garlic
5 tablespoons Greek yogurt
¼ cup red onion
½ cup cilantro
½ teaspoon salt
½ teaspoon pepper
¼ jalapeño (or ½ if you like it spicy)
2 tablespoons olive oil
¼ cup water (if sauce is too thick)

FOR THE TACOS

3 avocados
2 cups shredded green cabbage
8-16 corn or whole-wheat tortillas
Cilantro for garnish
Cotija cheese for garnish

METHOD

1. Peel and devein the shrimp. Pat them dry and season with cumin, black pepper, curry powder, turmeric, ground coriander, garlic powder, paprika, and salt.

2. Heat a pan on high and add olive oil. Once hot, add the shrimp. Reduce heat to medium-high and cook for 3-4 minutes until browned on one side, then flip and cook for another 3 minutes. Remove from the pan and set aside.

3. For the cilantro lime sauce, juice the limes into a blender. Add garlic, Greek yogurt, red onion, cilantro, salt, pepper, jalapeño, and olive oil. Blend for about a minute. Adjust consistency with water or more Greek yogurt as needed. Adjust seasoning to taste. Transfer sauce to a bottle or a plastic bag for drizzling.

4. Heat the tortillas in the same pan over medium heat for about a minute on each side.

5. Slice the avocados thinly.

6. Assemble the tacos: add avocado slices, shredded cabbage, and about 4 shrimp to each tortilla. Drizzle with cilantro lime sauce and garnish with Cotija cheese and cilantro.

7. Enjoy!

Total Servings	4
Per Serving	
Calories	613.5
Added Sugar	0g
Fiber	15.9g
Fat	31.5g
Saturated Fat	4.9g
Protein	30.15g

Values are estimated and can change according to ingredients used

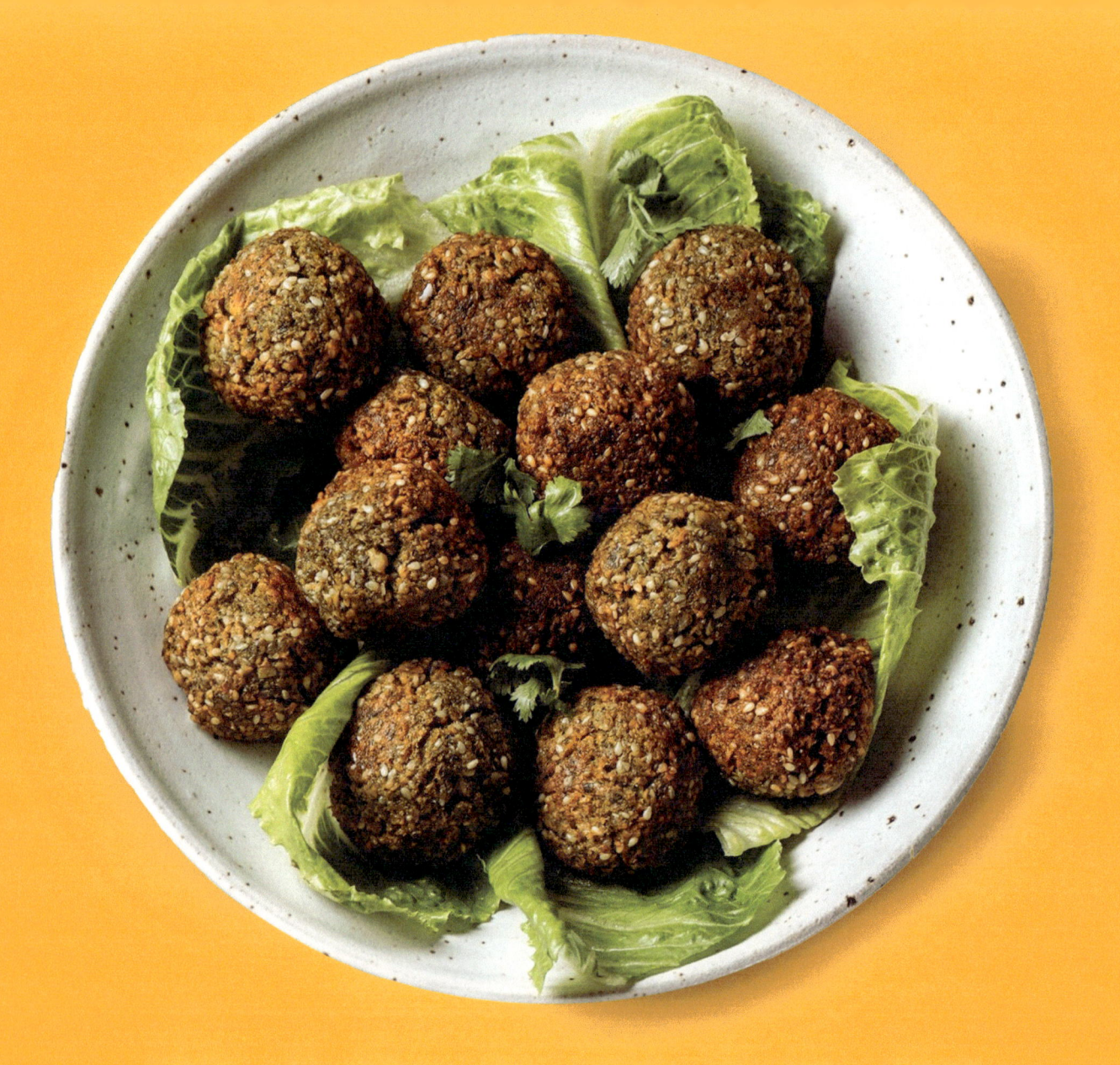

AIRFRIED FALAFEL

AIR-FRIED FALAFEL

Crunchy on the outside, soft on the inside, these air-fried falafels are a healthier take on a classic favorite.

INGREDIENTS

2 cups dried chickpeas (not canned)

1 cup white onion

2 cups parsley

2 cups cilantro

1 jalapeño

7 garlic cloves

2 teaspoons cumin

1 teaspoon coriander

1 teaspoon turmeric

1.5 tablespoons cornstarch

1.5 teaspoons baking powder

2 teaspoons salt

½ teaspoon black pepper

METHOD

1. Soak the chickpeas in water 24 hours before cooking. Ensure they are covered by about 3 inches of water.

2. After 24 hours, drain the chickpeas, which should have doubled or tripled in size.

3. Combine all ingredients in a food processor and pulse, scraping down the sides, until a paste forms.

4. Transfer the paste into a bowl. Form the mixture into balls, making 4-5 balls, depending on the size of your air fryer.

5. Brush all sides of the falafel balls with olive oil and place them in the air fryer.

6. Cook at 400°F for 5 minutes, or until the top half is browned. Flip the falafels, brush with olive oil, and cook for another 5 minutes at 400°F, or until uniformly browned.

7. Remove the falafels and serve with lemon tahini sauce or your favorite dipping sauce.

8. Enjoy!

Total Servings	4
Per Serving	
Calories	344.1
Added Sugar	0g
Fiber	13.1g
Fat	3.2g
Saturated Fat	0.3g
Protein	18.1g

Values are estimated and can change according to ingredients used

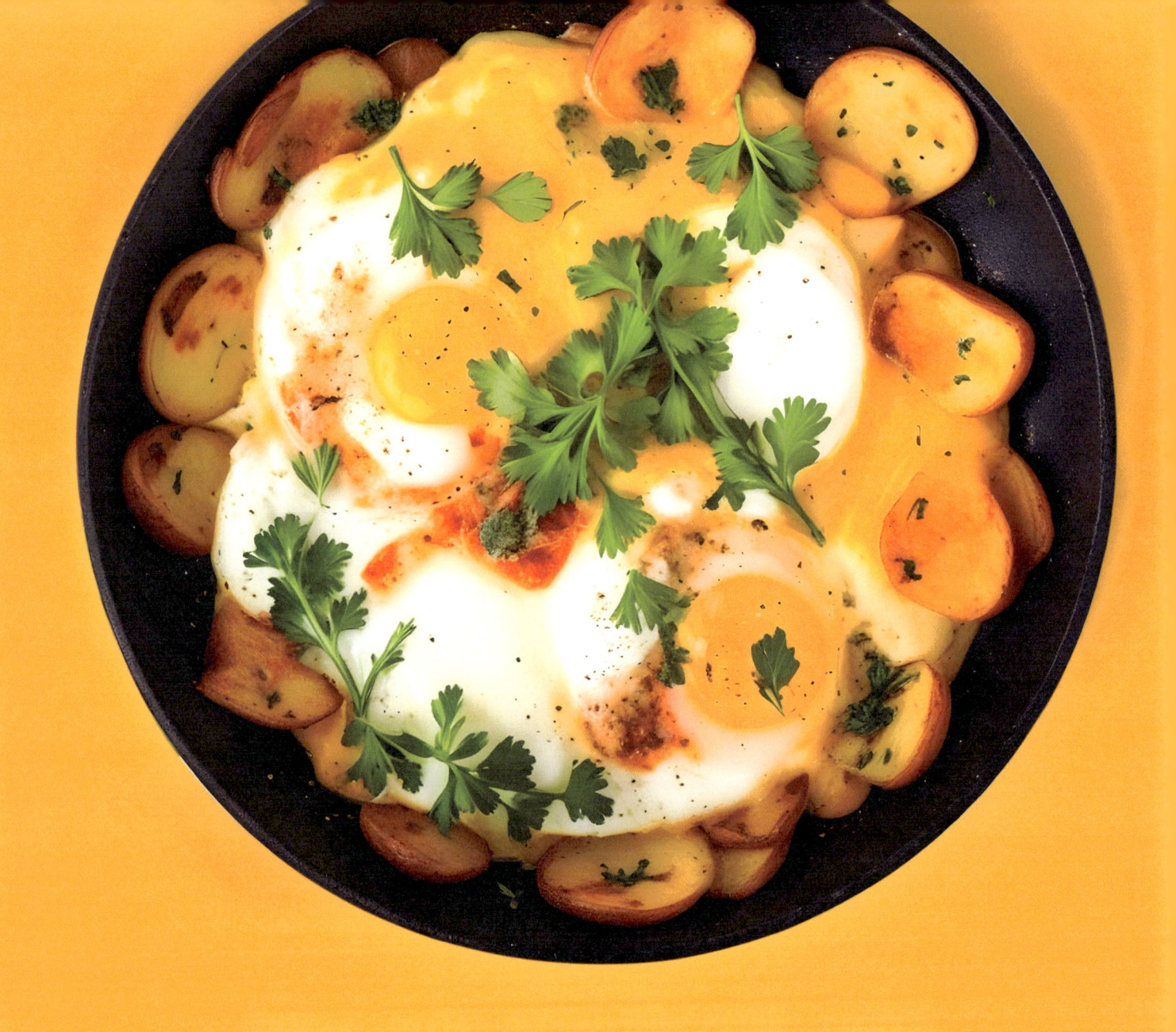

PAPETA PAR EEDA

PAPETA PAR EEDA

Meet your new favorite breakfast dish. Spiced potatoes and perfectly cooked eggs, all in one pan

INGREDIENTS

2 tablespoons olive oil

2 gold potatoes, sliced by mandolin (about 1 pound)

1 red onion, thinly sliced (about 1 pound)

3 Thai green chilies, thinly sliced (adjust to taste)

1 tablespoon ghee

3 cloves garlic, grated

1 tablespoon ginger, grated

¼ teaspoon cumin

¼ teaspoon turmeric

¼ cup cilantro

5 eggs

salt & pepper

Total Servings	5
Per Serving	
Calories	206.5
Added Sugar	0g
Fiber	2.4g
Fat	10.7g
Saturated Fat	3.3g
Protein	4.8g

Values are estimated and can change according to ingredients used

METHOD

1. Place the sliced potatoes in a bowl of cold water until needed.

2. Heat olive oil in a large saucepan over medium heat. Add the red onions and a pinch of salt. Cook for about 5 minutes, stirring constantly, until soft.

3. Add the garlic, ginger, and chilies. Cook for about 3 minutes, stirring constantly.

4. Add the ghee and drained potatoes. Stir in the cumin and turmeric.

5. Gently mix for a couple of minutes, then add the cilantro. Mix for another couple of minutes. Season to taste with salt and pepper.

6. Let the mixture cook undisturbed for about 10 minutes or until some potatoes are crispy.

7. Make 5 deep wells in the pan and crack an egg into each well. Reduce heat to low, cover the pan with a lid, and cook for 7 minutes.

8. Remove the lid. If the eggs are too runny, cook for an additional 1-2 minutes.

9. Serve and enjoy!

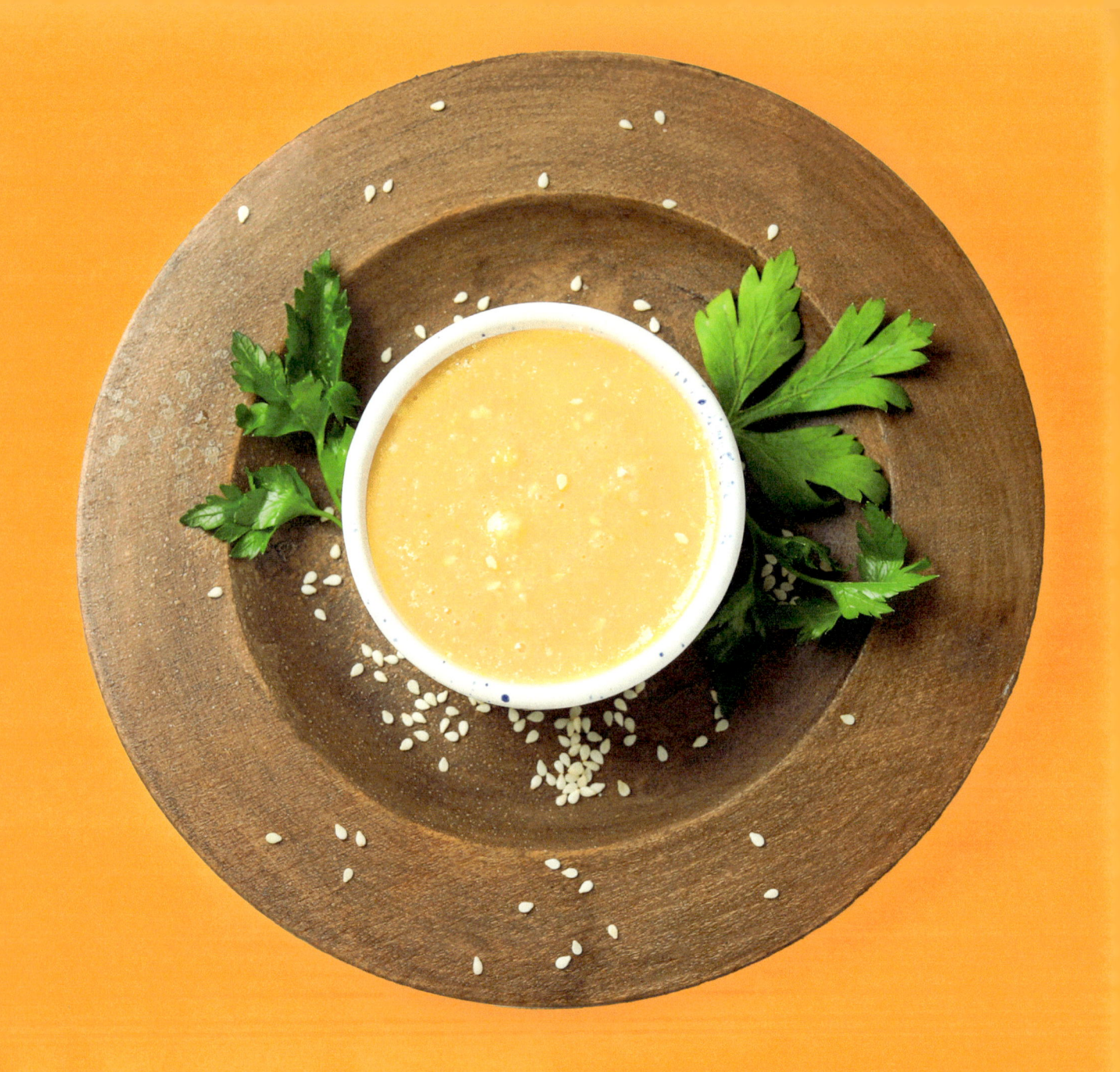

LEMON TAHINI SAUCE

LEMON TAHINI SAUCE

This lemon tahini sauce is the bomb. Tangy, nutty, and perfect on literally everything.

INGREDIENTS

¼ cup tahini

¼ cup lemon juice (about 1 lemon)

¾ tablespoon olive oil

Dash of honey

½ teaspoon salt

1 clove garlic, minced

Dash of cumin

Dash of turmeric

Dash of paprika

1.5 tablespoons water

METHOD

1. Combine all ingredients except the water in a small bowl and whisk together.

2. Slowly add the water while whisking until the sauce is creamy but not too thick. Adjust the amount of water to reach your desired consistency.

3. Enjoy this sauce with falafel, roasted vegetables, salads, or as a dip for fresh veggies.

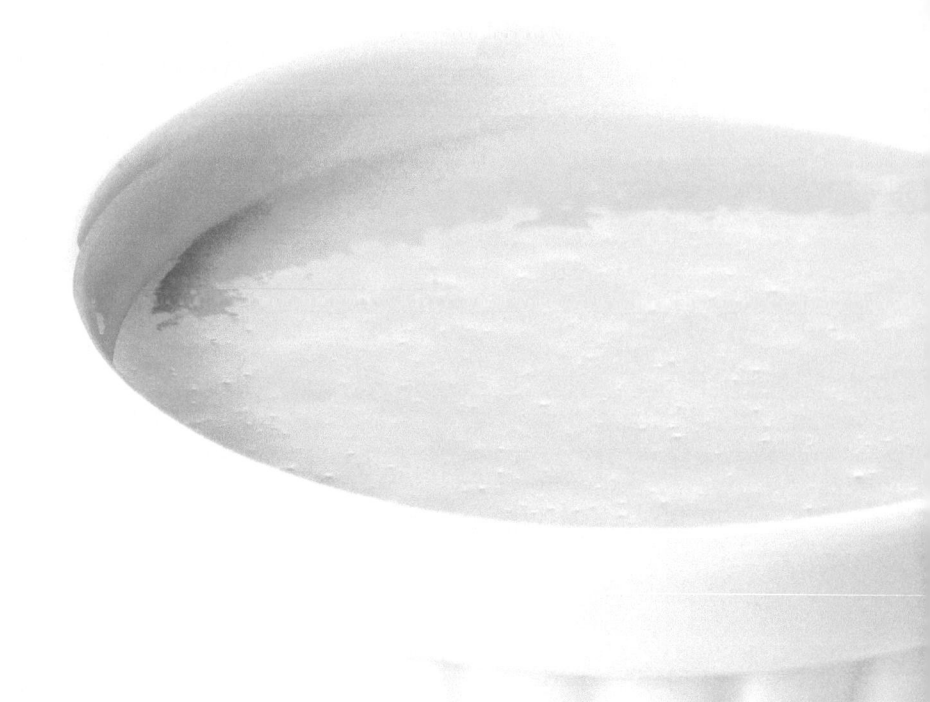

Total Servings	2
Per Serving	
Calories	152.5
Added Sugar	2.8g
Fiber	1.4g
Fat	13.1g
Saturated Fat	1.9g
Protein	2.7g

Values are approximate and may vary based on ingredients used

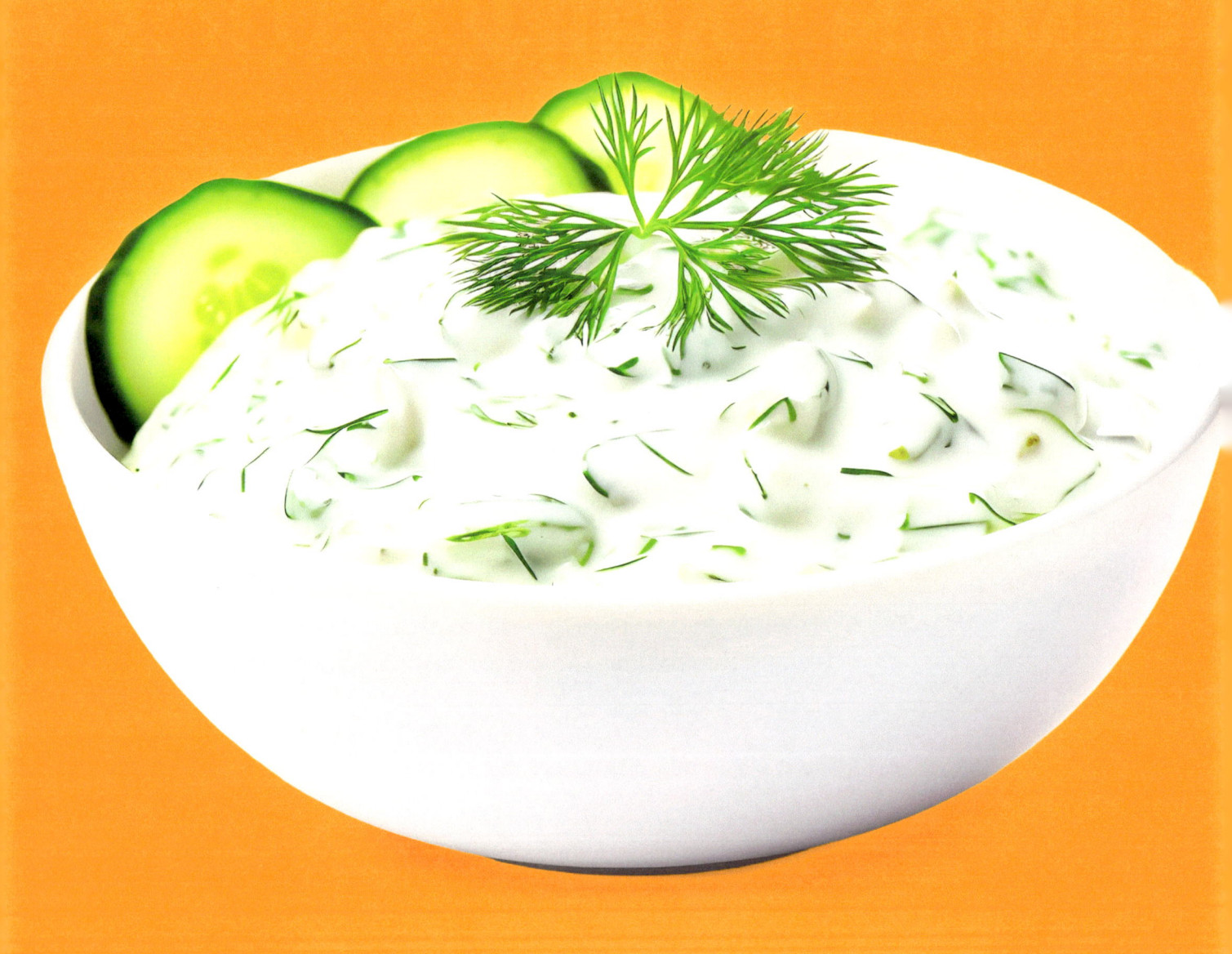

TZATZIKI SAUCE

TZATZIKI SAUCE

Cool, creamy, and refreshing—tzatziki is the ultimate sauce for dipping or topping your favorite dishes.

INGREDIENTS

¼ cup deseeded grated cucumber

½ cup non-fat Greek yogurt

½ tablespoon fresh lemon juice

¾ teaspoon olive oil

1 garlic clove, grated

Pinch of salt

½ tablespoon chopped fresh dill

METHOD

1. Squeeze the grated cucumber with a paper towel to remove excess liquid.

2. Combine all ingredients in a bowl and mix well.

3. Enjoy this sauce with grilled meats, gyros, pita bread, or as a dip for fresh vegetables.

Total Servings	2
Per Serving	
Calories	55.1
Added Sugar	0g
Fiber	0.2g
Fat	1.7g
Saturated Fat	0.25g
Protein	6.2g

Values are approximate and may vary based on ingredients used

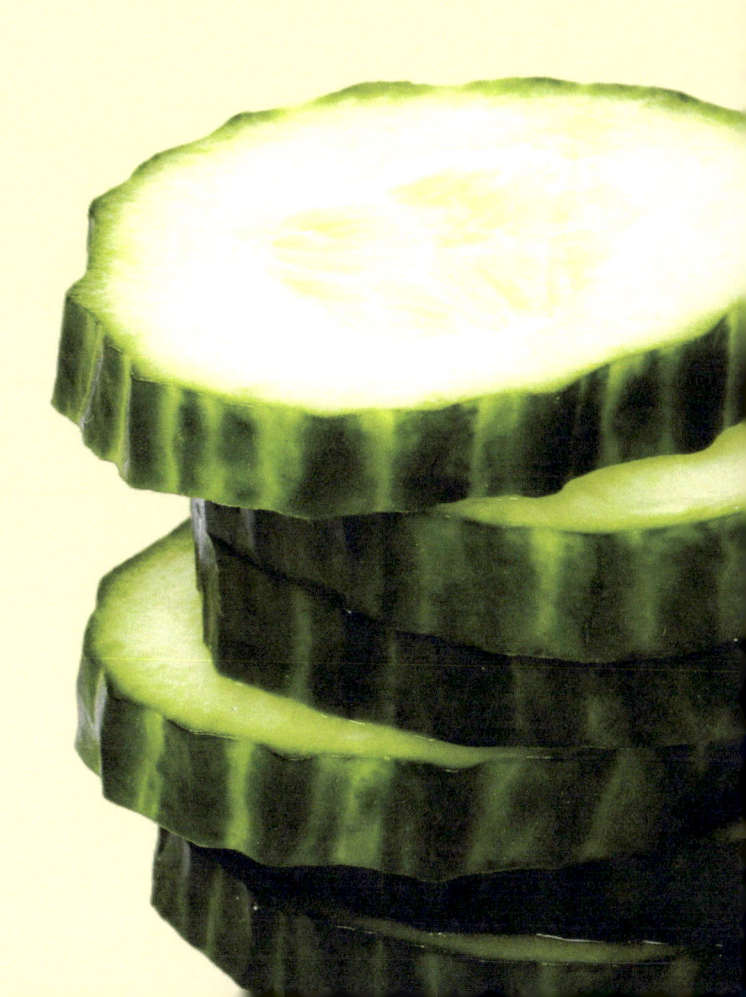

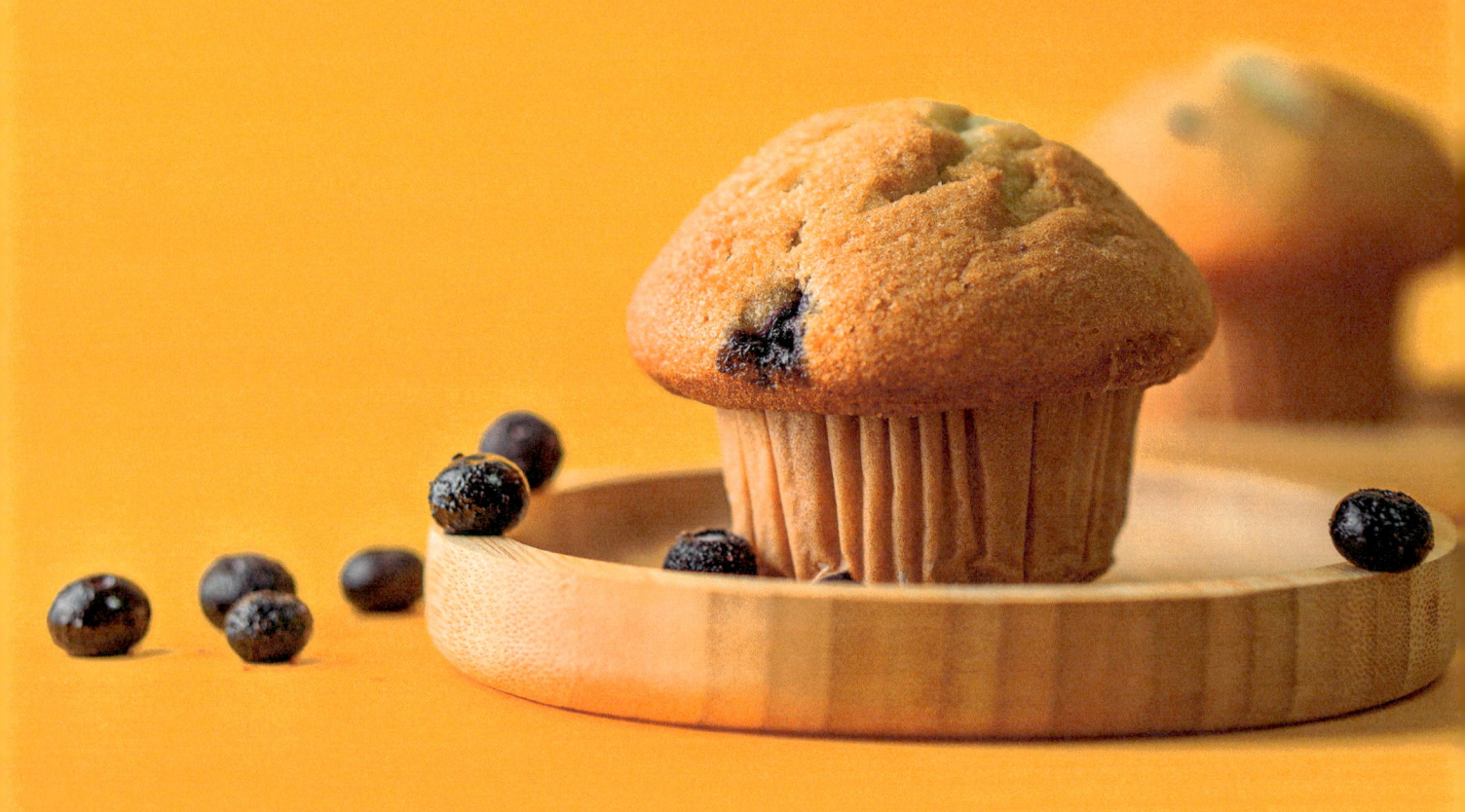

BLUEBERRY & APPLE MUFFIN

BLUEBERRY & APPLE MUFFINS

Start your day with these fruity and wholesome blueberry and apple muffins. Perfect for breakfast or a snack!

INGREDIENTS

1.5 cups whole-wheat flour

1 cup wheat bran

2.5 teaspoons baking powder

⅝ teaspoon baking soda (or ½ teaspoon and an extra pinch)

1.5 teaspoons ground cinnamon

¾ teaspoon ground nutmeg

¼ teaspoon salt

3 tablespoons canola oil

¼ cup non-fat Greek yogurt

¼ cup honey

2 eggs

2 teaspoons vanilla extract

1 cup non-fat milk

½ very sweet apple, blended

1 cup finely chopped red apples

1 cup blueberries

METHOD

1. Preheat the oven to 375°F (190°C).

2. In a bowl, whisk together flour, wheat bran, baking powder, baking soda, cinnamon, nutmeg, and salt.

3. Blend ½ of a very sweet apple until it is a liquid.

4. In a stand mixer or another bowl, beat together the oil, yogurt, and honey for 2 minutes until combined.

5. Beat in the eggs and vanilla until combined.

6. Slowly beat in the blended apple and mix for 2 minutes on low.

7. Gradually beat in half of the non-fat milk until combined, then add half of the dry ingredients and mix until combined.

8. Add the remaining non-fat milk and dry ingredients, mixing until fully combined.

9. Fold in the chopped apples and blueberries.

10. Pour the batter into muffin tray liners or a muffin tray sprayed with cooking spray.

11. Bake at 375°F for 20-25 minutes, or until a toothpick inserted into the center comes out clean.

12. Enjoy!

Total Servings	12
Per Serving	
Calories	123.3
Added Sugar	3.1g
Fiber	4.5g
Fat	2.8g
Saturated Fat	0.59g
Protein	4.9g

Values are approximate and may vary based on ingredients used

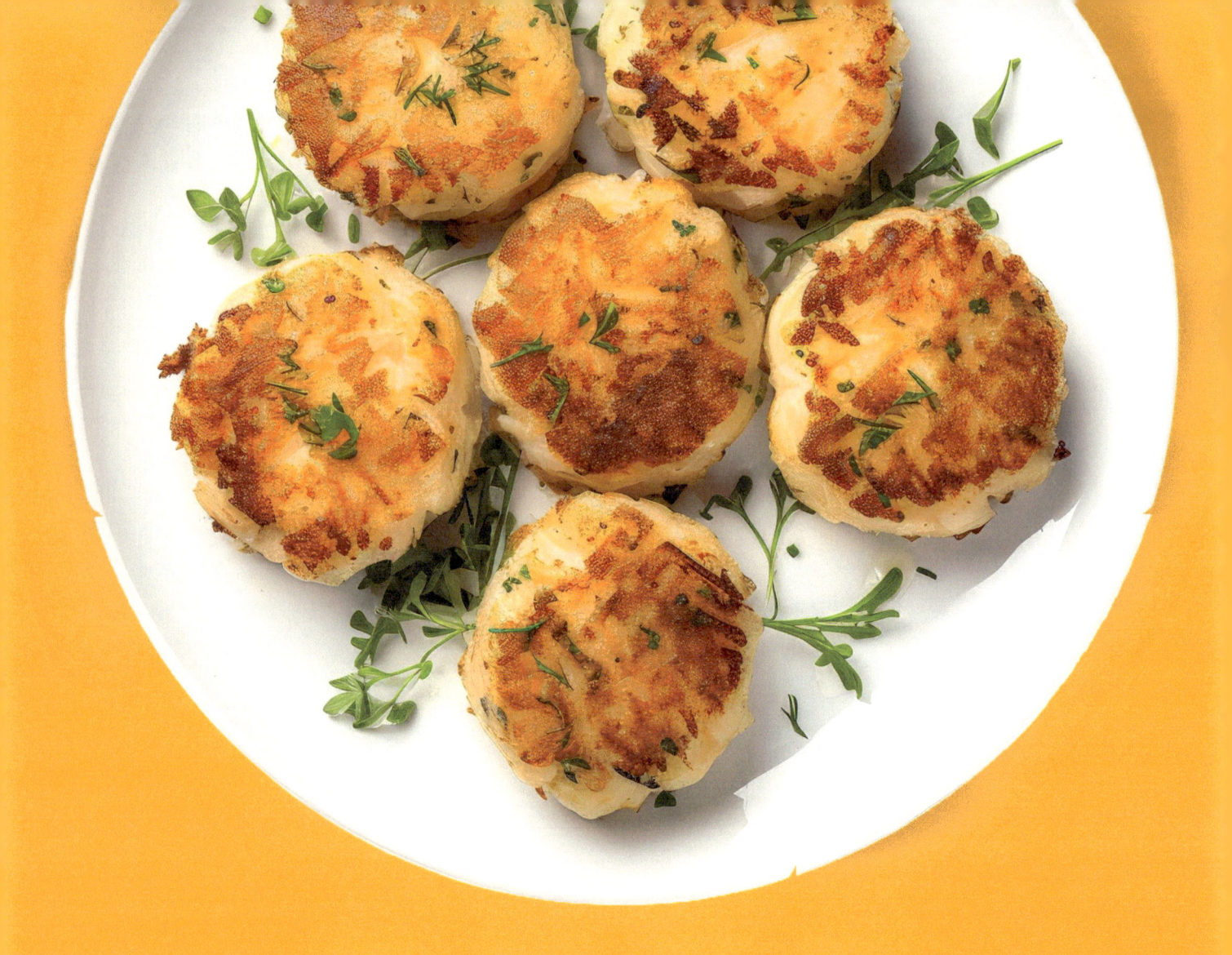

CRAB CAKES

CRAB CAKES

Treat yourself to these crispy, savory crab cakes. They're like a fancy restaurant dish you can make at home.

INGREDIENTS

1 egg

1 tablespoon non-fat Greek yogurt

1 teaspoon Dijon mustard

½ teaspoon Worcestershire sauce

½ teaspoon Old Bay seasoning

Pinch of salt

2 tablespoons finely diced celery stalks

1 tablespoon finely chopped parsley

8 oz lump crab meat

¼ cup whole-wheat panko bread crumbs

1 teaspoon olive oil

METHOD

1. Preheat the oven to 425°F (220°C).
2. In a bowl, combine all ingredients except the crab meat, panko, and olive oil.
3. Gently fold in the crab meat and panko until well combined.
4. Form the mixture into 5 crab cakes and place them on a baking sheet lined with parchment paper.
5. Refrigerate the crab cakes for 30 minutes to 1 hour.
6. Brush the top of each crab cake with olive oil.
7. Bake for about 25 minutes, or until the tops are nicely browned.
8. Remove from the oven and enjoy!

Total Servings	5
Per Serving	
Calories	67.3
Added Sugar	0.08g
Fiber	0.14g
Fat	2.4g
Saturated Fat	0.5g
Protein	8.4g

Values are approximate and may vary based on ingredients used

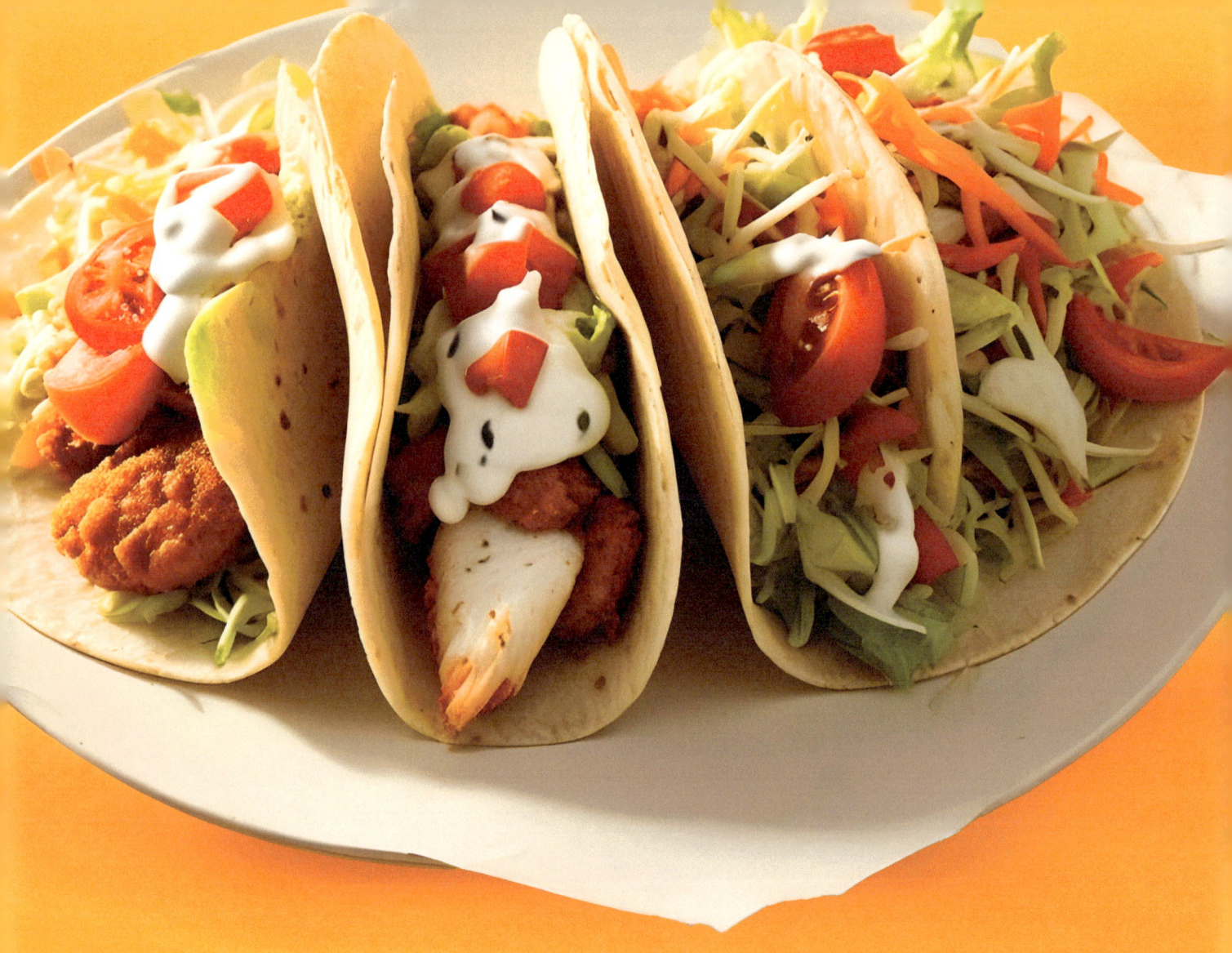

GRILLED FISH TACOS

GRILLED FISH TACOS

These fish tacos are next level. Topped with a tangy cilantro lime sauce and fresh veggies, they're a total win.

INGREDIENTS

FOR THE FISH

½ pound cod or any other white fish

⅛ teaspoon ground cumin

⅛ teaspoon cayenne

⅛ teaspoon garlic powder

⅛ teaspoon paprika

¼ teaspoon pepper

¼ teaspoon salt

¾ teaspoon olive oil

FOR THE SAUCE

½ cup cilantro

1.5 tablespoons non-fat Greek yogurt

½ jalapeño

Pinch of salt

¼ cup water

Juice of 1 lime

½ avocado

FOR THE TACOS

6 whole-wheat tortillas

¼ cup cabbage

½ avocado, sliced thin

1 Roma tomato, diced

¼ onion, diced

2 tablespoons cotija cheese

1 lime, cut into 6 slices

1 tablespoon cilantro

METHOD

1. Preheat the oven to 375°F (190°C).

2. Combine all sauce ingredients in a blender. Adjust the amount of water to achieve desired thickness. Pour into a sauce bottle.

3. Lay the fish on a baking sheet lined with parchment paper. Season both sides with cumin, cayenne, garlic powder, paprika, pepper, and salt. Drizzle with olive oil.

4. Bake the fish for 20 minutes. Remove from the oven and slice into 6 equal portions.

5. Toast tortillas on a hot pan for 1 minute on each side over high heat.

6. Assemble each taco: place one portion of fish on a tortilla, add avocado slices, cheese, cabbage, cilantro, onion, and tomato. Drizzle with sauce.

7. Serve with lime wedges and enjoy!

Total Servings	6
Per Serving	
Calories	160.2
Added Sugar	0g
Fiber	4.1g
Fat	4.8g
Saturated Fat	0.9g
Protein	12.4g

Values are approximate and may vary based on ingredients used

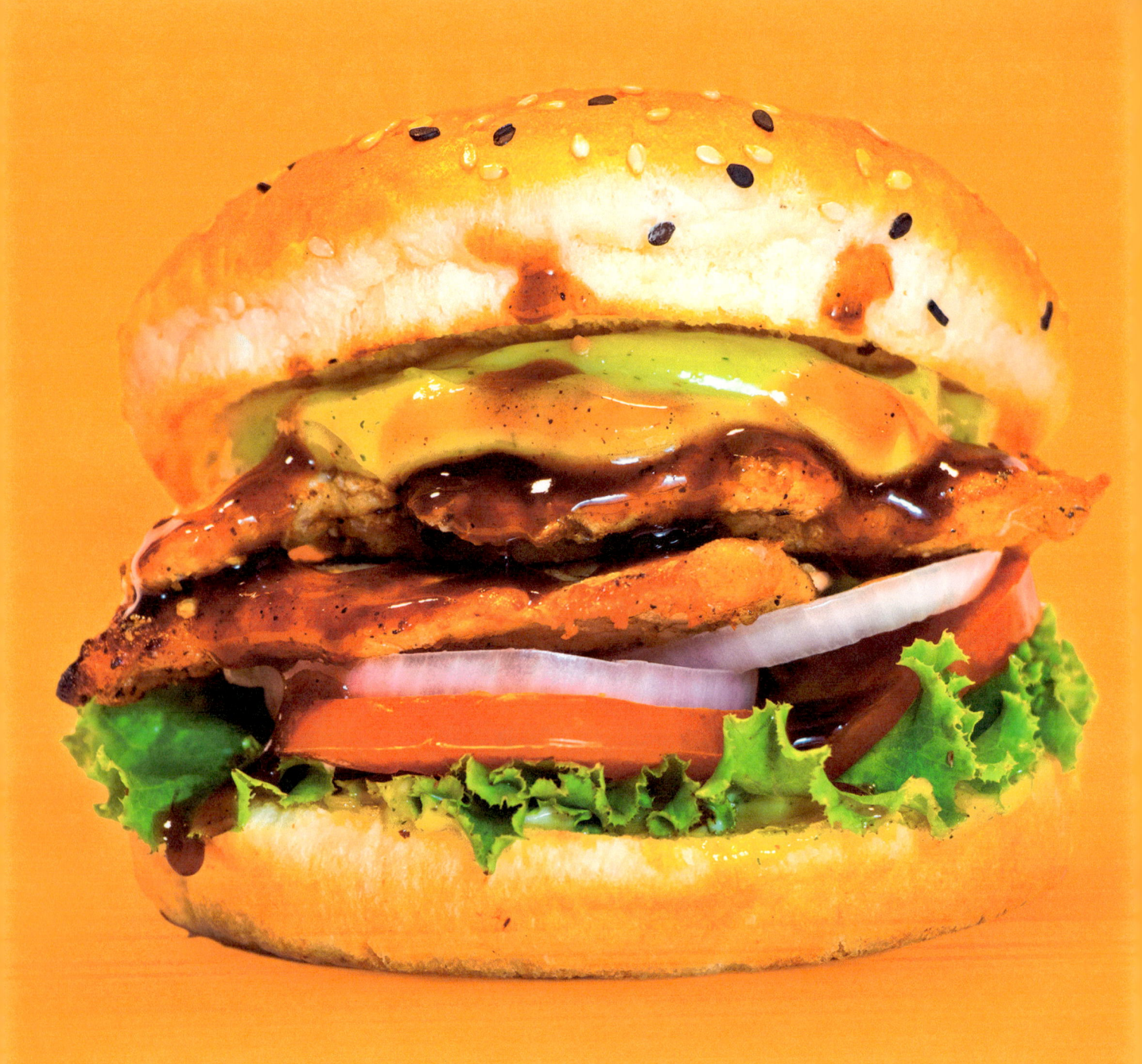

SPICY CHICKEN SANDWICH

SPICY CHICKEN SANDWICH

Turn up the heat with this spicy chicken sandwich. Crispy, juicy, and packed with flavor.

INGREDIENTS

2 chicken thighs

1.5 teaspoons salt

1.5 teaspoons pickle juice

½ teaspoon cumin

½ teaspoon cayenne pepper

Pinch of turmeric

1 teaspoon garlic powder

1 teaspoon buffalo hot sauce

2 tablespoons light ranch sauce (in this cookbook)

2 burger buns

½ cup cornflakes

½ cup all-purpose flour

½ cup crushed cornflakes

5 egg whites

6 pickle chips

METHOD

1. In a bowl, combine chicken thighs with salt, pickle juice, cumin, cayenne pepper, turmeric, garlic powder, and hot sauce. Marinate in the fridge for 30 minutes and up to overnight.

2. Prepare three bowls: one with crushed cornflakes, one with egg whites, and one with flour.

3. Fully coat the chicken in flour, then egg whites, and finally, crushed cornflakes. Ensure every part of the chicken is coated with cornflakes. Repeat for the other piece of chicken.

4. Spray your air fryer with cooking spray and place the coated chicken pieces inside. Cook at 380°F for 13-14 minutes, flipping halfway through, or until the internal temperature reaches 165°F.

5. While the chicken is cooking, toast the buns in a toaster.

6. Spread 1 tablespoon of light ranch sauce on the bottom halves of each bun. Add 3 pickle chips to each bun.

7. Once the chicken is done, place one piece on each bun to make two sandwiches.

8. Enjoy!

Total Servings	2
Per Serving	
Calories	525.5
Added Sugar	4.3g
Fiber	2.5g
Fat	13.8g
Saturated Fat	3.5g
Protein	29.3g

Values are approximate and may vary based on ingredients used

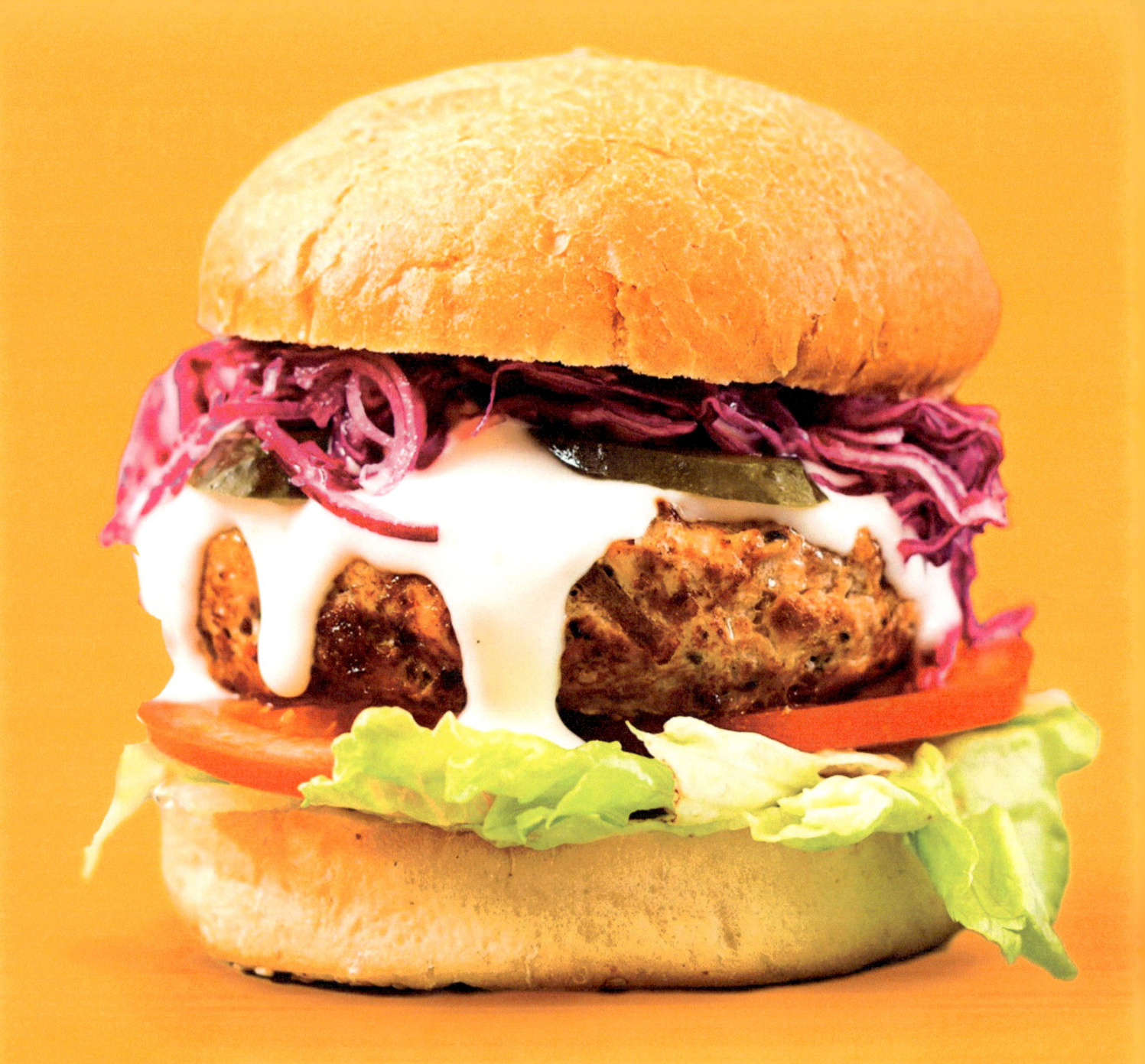

CHICKEN SANDWICH

CHICKEN SANDWICH

Classic chicken sandwich vibes. Crispy on the outside, juicy on the inside, and totally satisfying.

INGREDIENTS

2 chicken thighs

1.5 teaspoons salt

1.5 teaspoons pickle juice

¼ teaspoon cumin

Pinch of turmeric

1 teaspoon garlic powder

1 teaspoon buffalo hot sauce

2 tablespoons light ranch sauce (see cookbook)

2 burger buns

½ cup cornflakes

½ cup all-purpose flour

½ cup crushed cornflakes

5 egg whites

6 pickle chips

METHOD

1. In a bowl, combine chicken thighs with salt, pickle juice, cumin, turmeric, garlic powder, and hot sauce. Marinate in the fridge for 30 minutes and up to overnight.

2. Prepare three bowls: one with crushed cornflakes, one with egg whites, and one with flour.

3. Fully coat the chicken in flour, then egg whites, and finally, crushed cornflakes. Ensure every part of the chicken is coated with cornflakes. Repeat for the other piece of chicken.

4. Spray your air fryer with cooking spray and place the coated chicken pieces inside. Cook at 380°F for 13-14 minutes, flipping halfway through, or until the internal temperature reaches 165°F.

5. While the chicken is cooking, toast the buns in a toaster.

6. Spread 1 tablespoon of light ranch sauce on the bottom halves of each bun. Add 3 pickle chips to each bun.

7. Once the chicken is done, place one piece on each bun to make two sandwiches.

8. Enjoy!

Total Servings	2
Per Serving	
Calories	523
Added Sugar	4.3g
Fiber	2.35g
Fat	13.7g
Saturated Fat	3.5g
Protein	29.2g

Values are approximate and may vary based on ingredients used

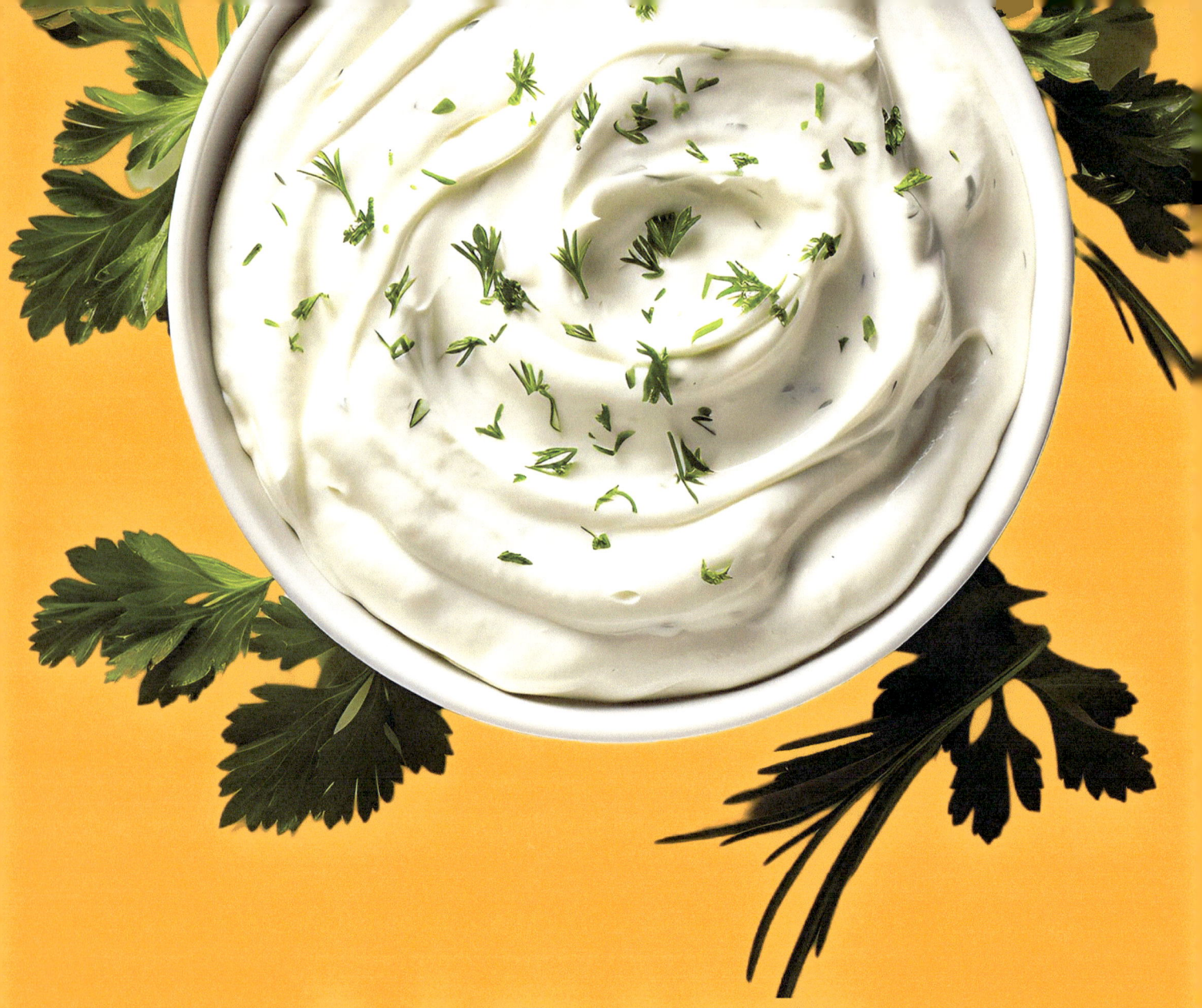

LIGHT RANCH

LIGHT RANCH

All the creamy, herby goodness of ranch dressing, but lighter. Perfect on salads, veggies, and more!

INGREDIENTS

½ cup non-fat Greek yogurt

½ teaspoon fresh chopped dill

½ teaspoon fresh chopped chives

½ teaspoon Worcestershire sauce

1 teaspoon buffalo hot sauce

½ teaspoon white distilled vinegar

Salt to taste

METHOD

1. Combine all ingredients except for the salt in a bowl and mix well.

2. Add salt to taste.

3. Enjoy!

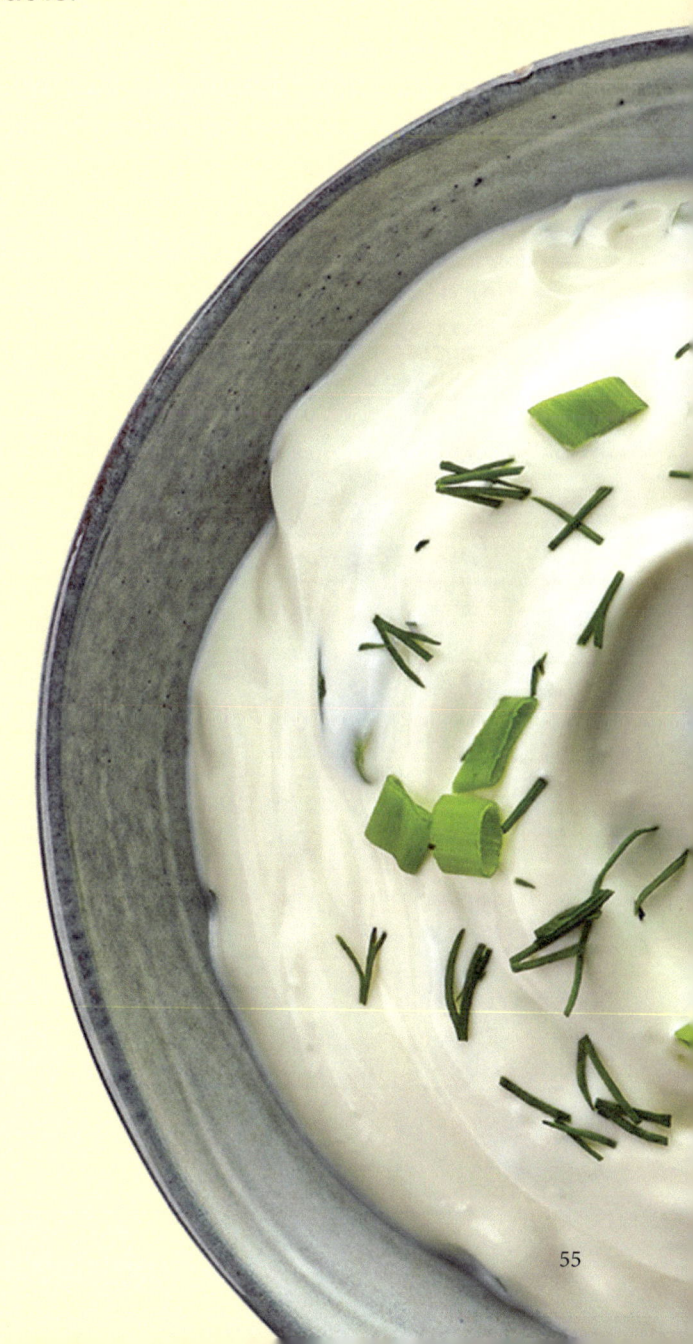

Total Servings	2
Per Serving	
Calories	34
Added Sugar	0.15g
Fiber	0.15g
Fat	0.15g
Saturated Fat	0.05g
Protein	5.5g

Values are approximate and may vary based on ingredients used

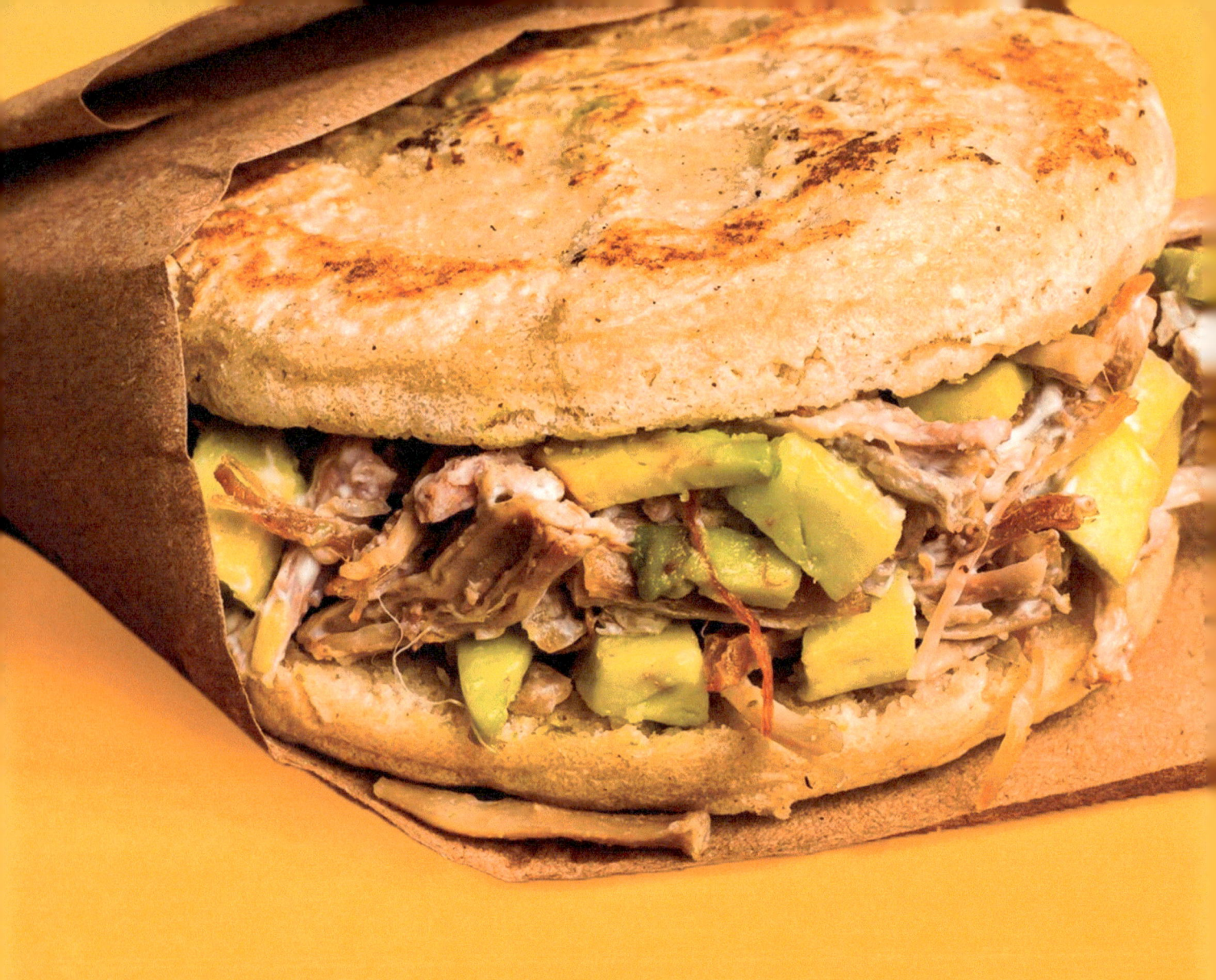

BREAKFAST SANDWICH

BREAKFAST SANDWICH

Start your morning with this hearty breakfast sandwich. It's packed with protein and flavor.

INGREDIENTS

½ pound 95% lean ground beef

1 dried guajillo chili, seeds removed

1 dried ancho chili, seeds removed

1 large garlic clove

1.5 tablespoons distilled white vinegar

1 teaspoon cumin

1 teaspoon salt

½ teaspoon ground coriander seeds

¼ teaspoon onion powder

Dash of cinnamon

1 teaspoon olive oil

8 egg whites

2 slices low-fat American cheese

Pinch of salt

½ avocado, sliced thin

½ large tomato, diced

¼ white onion, diced

½ tablespoon cilantro leaves, chopped

½ teaspoon lime zest

Juice from 1 lime

2 whole-wheat tortillas

METHOD

1. Boil water and add dried chilis. Cook until soft. Remove from water and blend with garlic, vinegar, cumin, salt, coriander, onion powder, and cinnamon. Add chili water gradually until smooth.

2. Combine ground beef with the blended sauce in a bowl. Mix until well combined. Use immediately or marinate overnight in the fridge.

3. Heat a non-stick skillet over medium-high heat. Cook the meat until thoroughly browned, about 6 minutes. Set aside.

4. In a bowl, combine diced tomato, diced onion, cilantro leaves, lime zest, and lime juice. Mix well. Set aside.

5. Heat olive oil in a non-stick pan over medium heat. Add egg whites and cheese, and a pinch of salt. Stir constantly until creamy.

6. Lay out a whole-wheat tortilla. Add half the cooked meat mixture, half the eggs, pico de gallo, and half the avocado slices. Repeat for the second tortilla.

7. Wrap the tortillas tightly.

8. Enjoy!

Total Servings	2
Per Serving	
Calories	474.5
Added Sugar	0g
Fiber	10.1g
Fat	17.8g
Saturated Fat	4.1g
Protein	41.1g

Values are approximate and may vary based on ingredients used

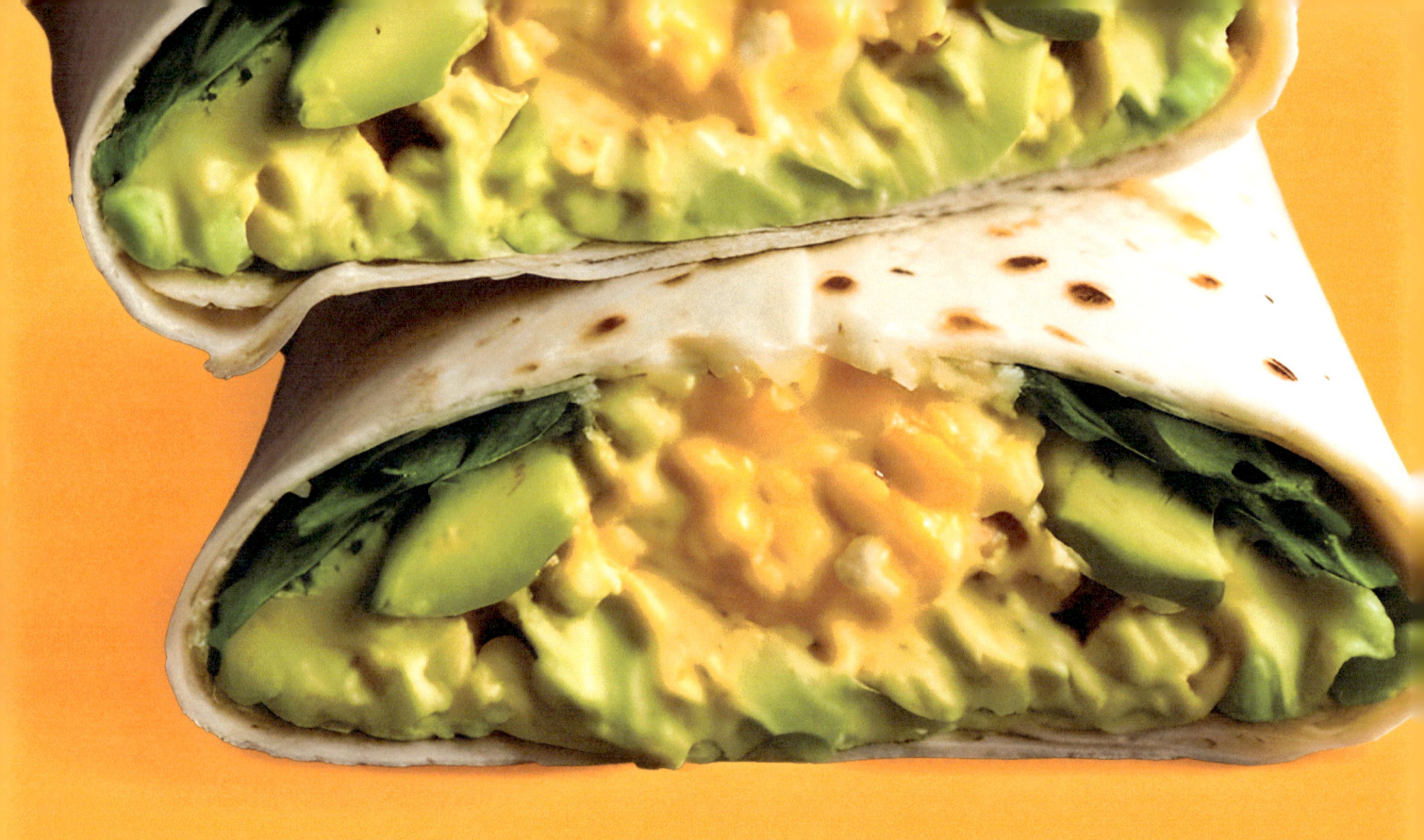

MY DAD'S FAVORITE BREAKFAST SANDWICH

MY DAD'S FAVORITE BREAKFAST SANDWICH

This breakfast sandwich is my dad's fave. Fluffy eggs, creamy avocado crema, and crispy red onions—what's not to love?

INGREDIENTS

1 whole-wheat tortilla

2 eggs, whisked

4 thin slices of red onion

1 slice low-fat American cheese

½ tablespoon avocado crema

1 teaspoon olive oil

METHOD

1. Heat olive oil in a pan over medium-high heat.
2. Once hot, add the whisked eggs. Cook for 30 seconds, stirring constantly.
3. Add the American cheese and cook for another 30 seconds to a minute, until eggs are done.
4. Place the cooked eggs, avocado crema, and red onion slices on the tortilla.
5. Wrap it up.
6. Enjoy!

Total Servings	1
Per Serving	
Calories	340.5
Added Sugar	0g
Fiber	3.9g
Fat	18.6g
Saturated Fat	5.2g
Protein	18.9g

Values are approximate and may vary based on ingredients used

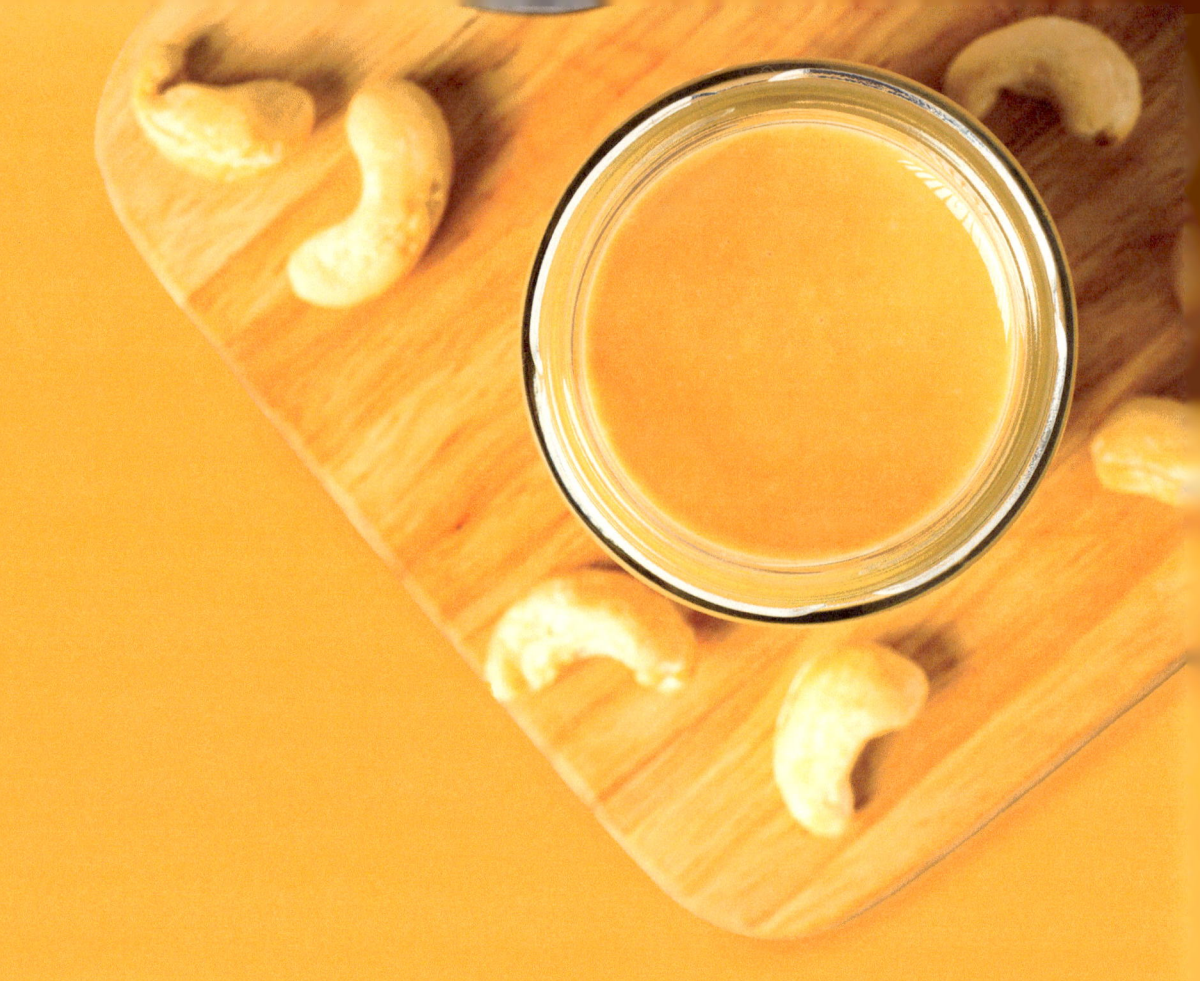

CAESAR SALAD DRESSING

CAESAR SALAD DRESSING

Upgrade your salads with this creamy, tangy Caesar dressing. It's got a secret ingredient that makes it extra yummy!

INGREDIENTS

1 cup raw unsalted cashews

2 teaspoons anchovy paste

½ cup water

¼ cup lemon juice

2 teaspoons nutritional yeast

1 clove garlic

METHOD

1. Put cashews in a pot, cover with water, and bring to a boil. Boil for 8 minutes.

2. After boiling, drain the cashews and add them to a blender with the rest of the ingredients.

3. Blend until very smooth. Adjust consistency by adding more cashews if too thin or more water if too thick.

4. Season to taste.

5. Enjoy!

Total Servings	2
Per Serving	
Calories	418.2
Added Sugar	0g
Fiber	2.65g
Fat	32.6g
Saturated Fat	6.5g
Protein	16.1g

Values are approximate and may vary based on ingredients used

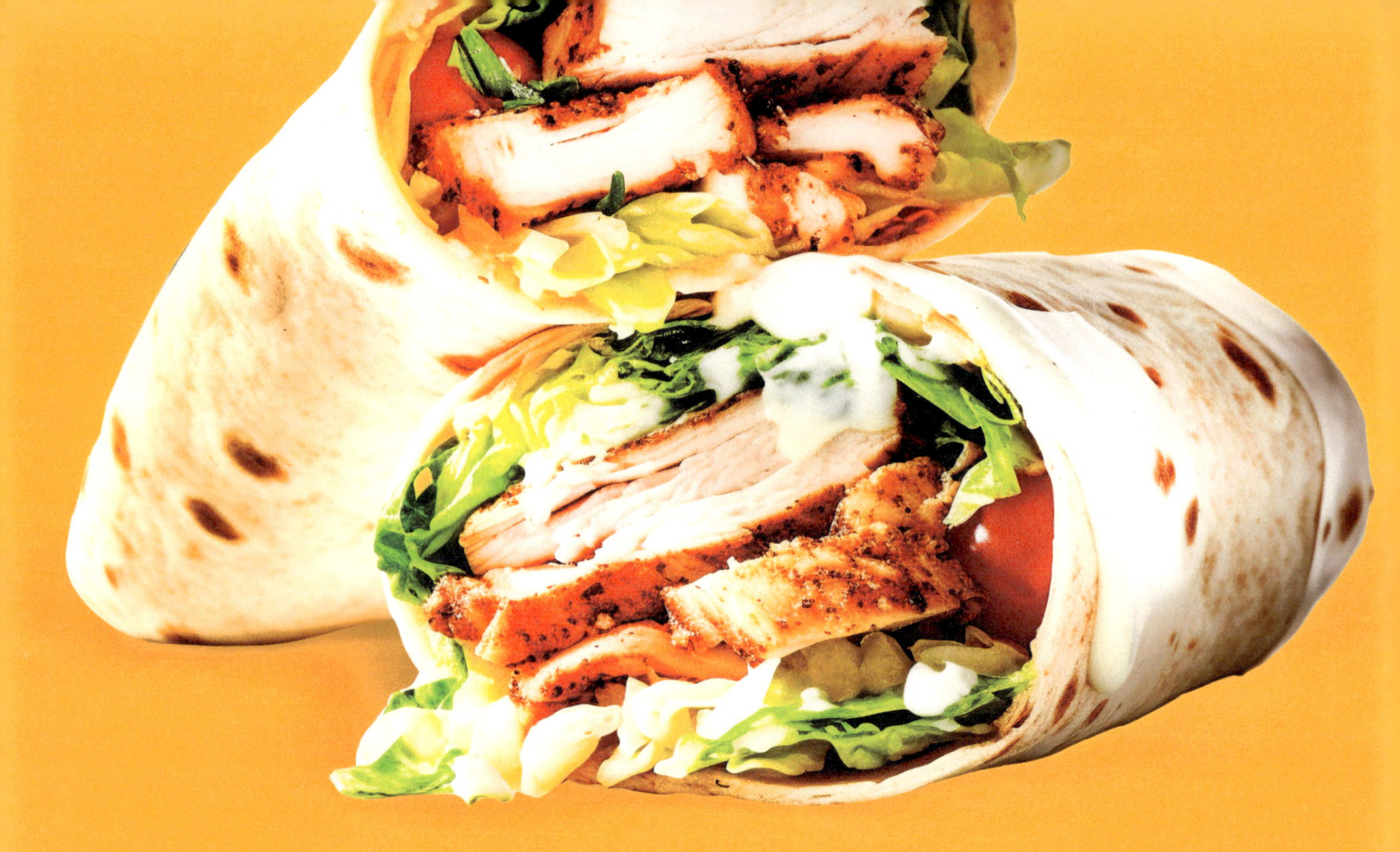

CHICKEN CAESAR WRAP

CHICKEN CAESAR WRAP

All the classic Caesar salad flavors wrapped up in a convenient, delicious wrap. Perfect for lunch on the go!

INGREDIENTS

4 chicken breasts

7 oz chipotle peppers in adobo

5 cloves garlic

½ cup water

2 teaspoons salt

1 teaspoon olive oil

Dash of turmeric

Dash of cumin

4 whole-wheat wraps

4 cups romaine lettuce

Caesar Salad Dressing (see recipe)

METHOD

1. Combine chipotle peppers in adobo, garlic, water, salt, turmeric, and cumin in a blender until smooth.

2. Marinate the chicken breasts in the blended mixture for at least 30 minutes or up to overnight in the fridge.

3. Heat olive oil in a pan over medium-high heat. Cook the chicken breasts for 2-3 minutes on each side or until the internal temperature reaches 165°F. Remove from the pan and let rest for 5-10 minutes.

4. Once rested, cut the chicken into thin cubes.

5. In a bowl, combine the cubed chicken with 1 cup of romaine lettuce and about a tablespoon of Caesar salad dressing.

6. Toast a whole-wheat wrap in the same pan for a minute on each side. Remove from the pan.

7. Add the chicken and lettuce mixture to the wrap. Wrap it up tightly.

8. Repeat for the remaining wraps.

9. Enjoy!

Total Servings	4
Per Serving	
Calories	280.8
Added Sugar	0g
Fiber	6.3g
Fat	5.25g
Saturated Fat	1.08g
Protein	29.1g

Values are approximate and don't include dressing.

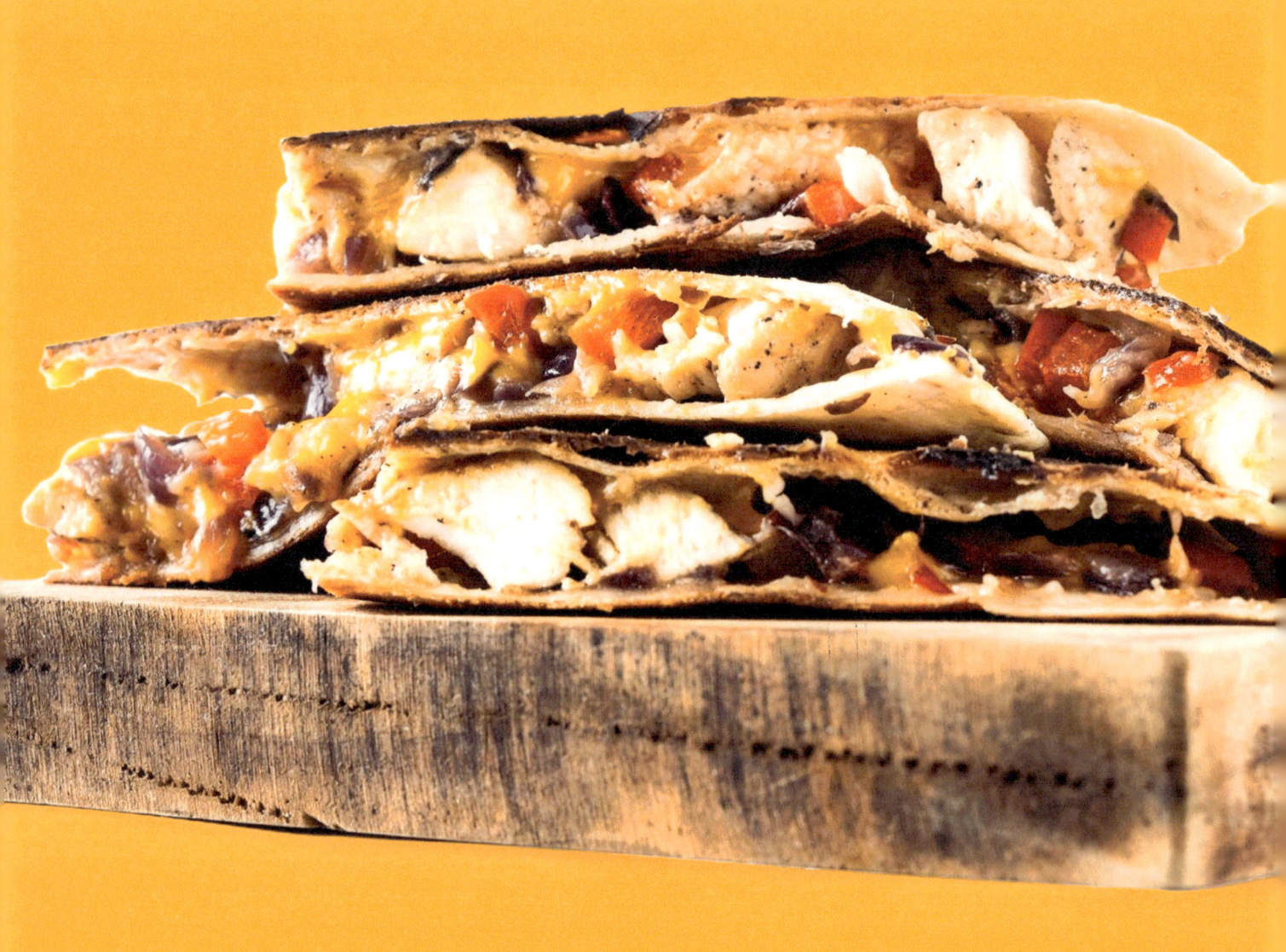

CHICKEN QUESADILLAS

CHICKEN QUESADILLAS

Cheesy, flavorful chicken quesadillas that hit the spot every time. Quick, easy, and super tasty.

INGREDIENTS

- 4 chicken breasts
- 7 oz chipotle peppers in adobo
- 5 cloves garlic
- ½ cup water
- 2 teaspoons salt
- 1 teaspoon olive oil
- Dash of turmeric
- Dash of cumin
- Dash of paprika
- 15 oz can of corn
- 1 jalapeño, diced
- 1.5 tablespoons diced red onion
- 1.5 tablespoons chopped cilantro
- 2 large cloves garlic, grated
- 1 cup shredded low-fat mozzarella cheese
- 1 cup shredded low-fat cheddar cheese
- 4 whole-wheat tortillas

METHOD

1. Combine chipotle peppers in adobo, garlic, water, salt, turmeric, cumin, and paprika in a blender until smooth.
2. Marinate the chicken breasts in the blended mixture for at least 30 minutes or up to overnight in the fridge.
3. In a bowl, mix the corn, jalapeño, onion, cilantro, and grated garlic.
4. Heat olive oil in a pan over medium-high heat. Cook the chicken breasts for 2-3 minutes on each side or until the internal temperature reaches 165°F. Remove from the pan and let rest for 5-10 minutes.
5. Once rested, cut the chicken into thin cubes.
6. On the same pan over medium heat, lay out a tortilla. Add a tablespoon each of mozzarella and cheddar cheese to one side, some chicken, and a tablespoon of the corn mixture.
7. Fold the tortilla in half and cook for another minute on each side, until the cheese is melted and the tortilla is golden brown.
8. Remove from the pan and repeat with the remaining tortillas.
9. Enjoy!

Total Servings	4
Per Serving	
Calories	399.1
Added Sugar	0g
Fiber	7.3g
Fat	10.4g
Saturated Fat	4.1g
Protein	38g

Values are approximate and may vary based on ingredients used

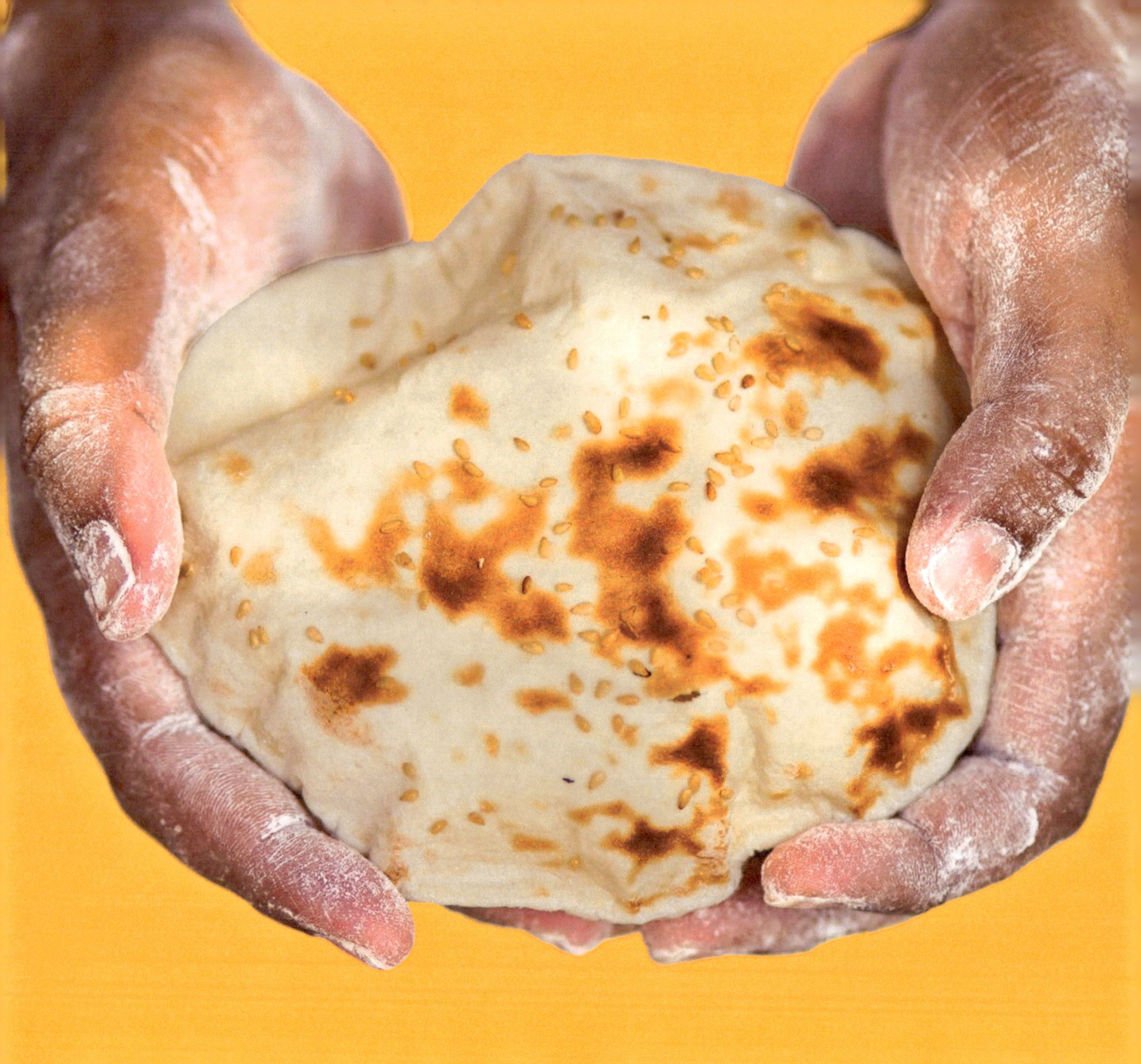

WHOLE WHEAT TORTILLAS

WHOLE-WHEAT TORTILLAS

Homemade whole-wheat tortillas add a hearty, nutty flavor to your wraps, tacos, and quesadillas.

INGREDIENTS

2 cups whole-wheat flour

⅔ teaspoon baking powder

1 teaspoon salt

2 tablespoons vegetable oil

1 cup boiling water

METHOD

1. In a bowl, combine whole-wheat flour, baking powder, and salt.

2. Add vegetable oil and mix until well combined.

3. Pour in boiling water and mix with a wooden spoon until cool enough to handle. Form into a dough and knead until smooth.

4. Divide the dough into 8 equal pieces and shape them into balls.

5. Flatten each ball into a thick disk.

6. Cover the disks with a damp towel and let them rest for 20 minutes.

7. After resting, dust both sides of a disk with whole-wheat flour.

8. Roll out the dough into a thin 8-inch tortilla.

9. Heat a pan over high heat. Cook the tortilla for 1 minute on each side until bubbles form.

10. Place cooked tortillas in a bowl and cover with a lid to keep them warm.

11. Repeat for all tortillas.

12. Enjoy!

Total Servings	8
Per Serving	
Calories	144.1
Added Sugar	0g
Fiber	4.5g
Fat	4g
Saturated Fat	0.7g
Protein	4.08g

Values are approximate and may vary based on ingredients used

MANGO FRUIT LEATHER

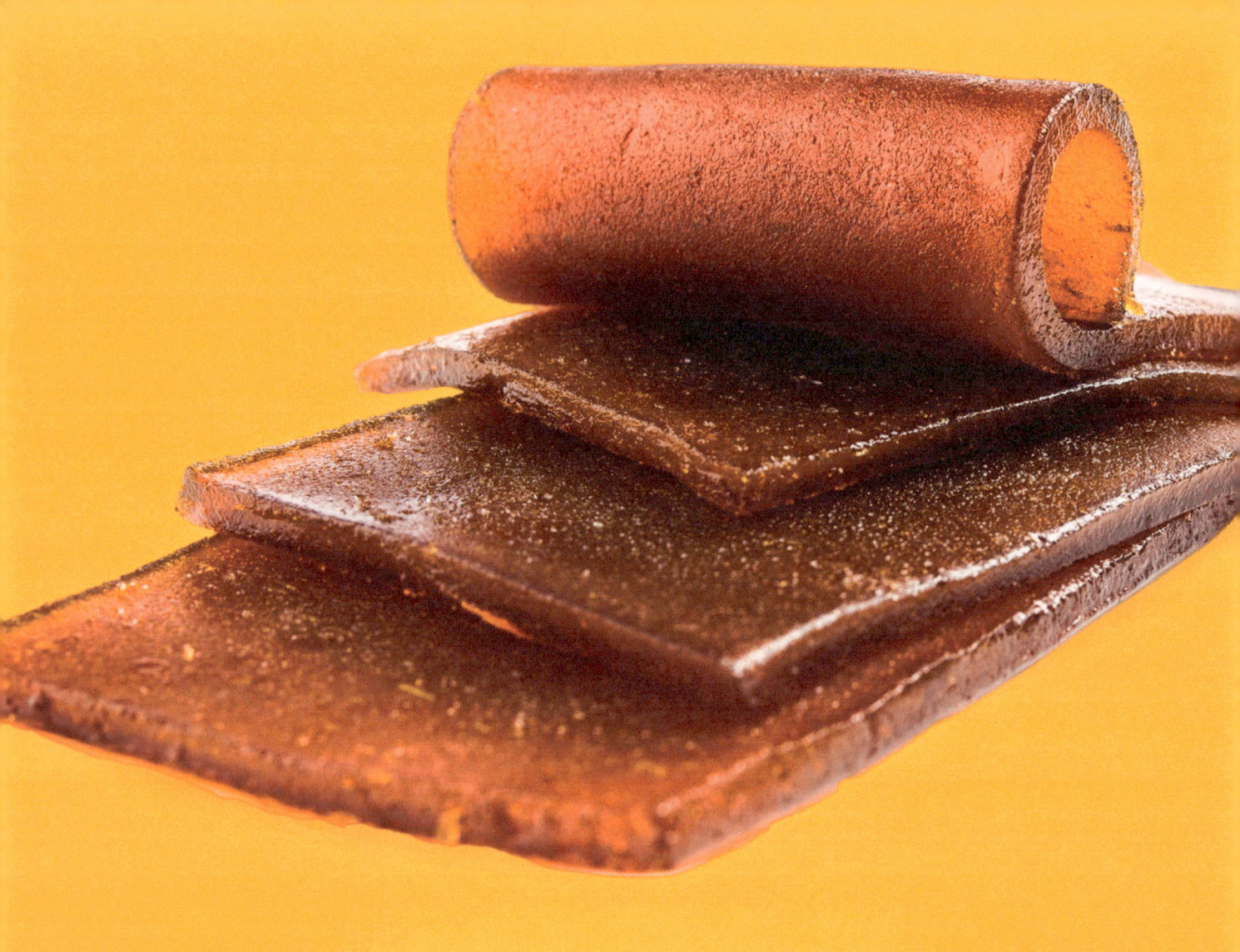

MANGO FRUIT LEATHER

Homemade mango fruit leather is a sweet and tangy snack that's perfect anytime. So easy to make!

INGREDIENTS

1 pound mangoes

1 teaspoon lemon juice

1 teaspoon water

1 teaspoon honey

METHOD

1. Preheat oven to 170°F (75°C).
2. Peel and deseed the mangoes. Add them to a blender along with the honey, lemon juice, and water.
3. Blend until very smooth.
4. Pour the blended mixture onto a parchment-lined baking sheet, spreading it as flat and thin as possible.
5. Bake in the oven for 4 hours, or until the fruit leather is dry to the touch and no longer sticky.
6. Remove from the oven and let it cool.
7. Enjoy!

Total Servings	8
Per Serving	
Calories	19.8
Added Sugar	0.7g
Fiber	0.6g
Fat	0.1g
Saturated Fat	0.03g
Protein	0.1g

Values are approximate and may vary based on ingredients used

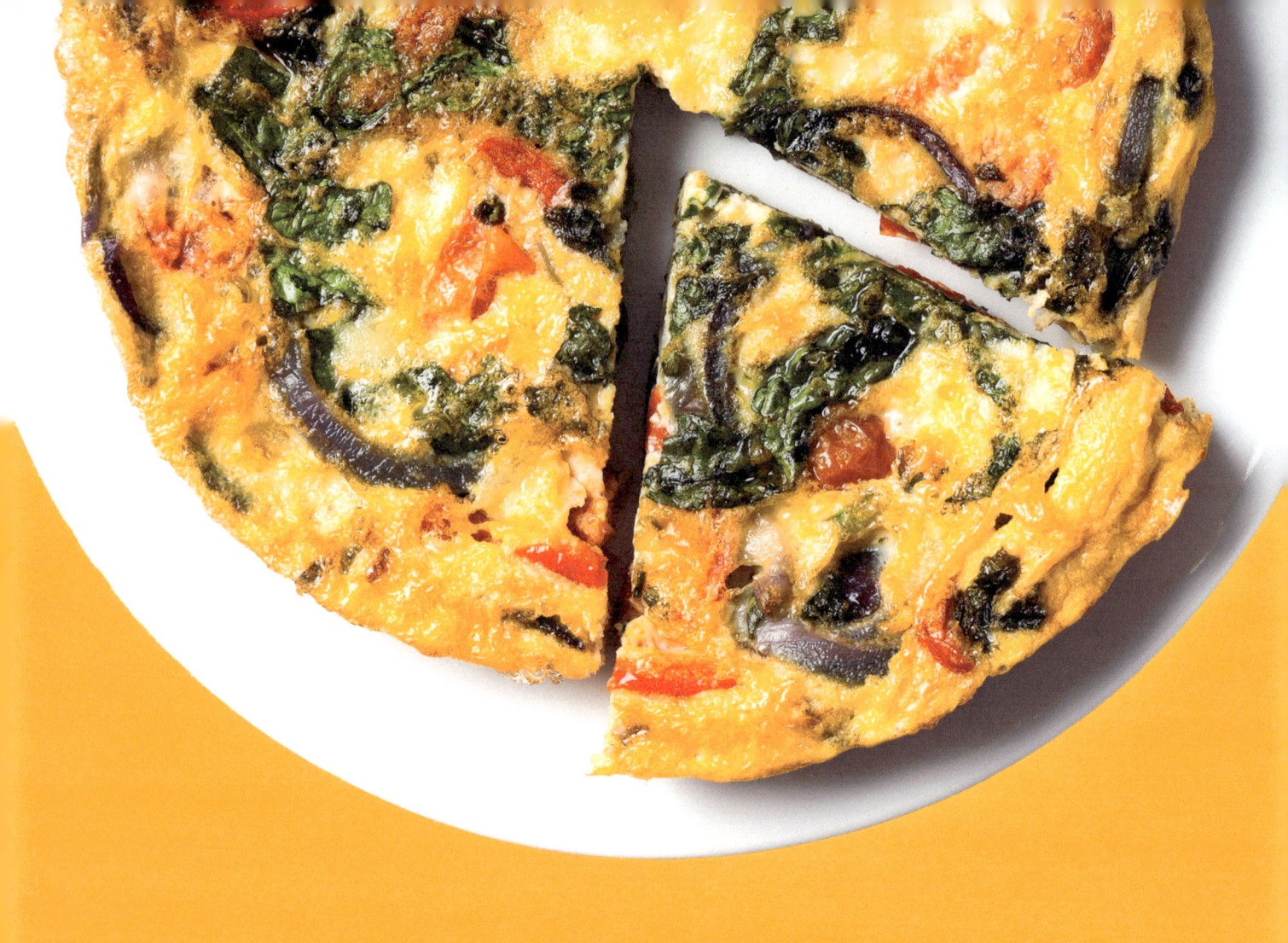

CRUSTLESS QUICHE

CRUSTLESS QUICHE

This light and fluffy crustless quiche is loaded with veggies and cheese. Perfect for breakfast or brunch.

INGREDIENTS

1 red onion, thinly sliced

1.5 teaspoons olive oil

1 teaspoon salt (for onions)

5 spinach leaves, chopped thin

4 medium white mushrooms, chopped thin

1 cup shredded cheese (Gruyere, cheddar, Swiss, Parmesan, or Gouda)

½ cup all-purpose flour

¾ teaspoon baking powder

1.5 cups non-fat milk

4 large eggs, whisked

2.5 teaspoons Dijon mustard

½ teaspoon salt

½ teaspoon pepper

Total Servings	6
Per Serving	
Calories	195
Added Sugar	0g
Fiber	0.9g
Fat	10.5g
Saturated Fat	5g
Protein	11.6g

Values are approximate and may vary based on ingredients used

METHOD

1. Preheat oven to 375°F (190°C).

2. Heat olive oil in a pan over medium-high heat. Add the red onion, reduce heat to low, and season with 1 teaspoon salt. Cook for 8-10 minutes, stirring occasionally, until soft and translucent.

3. Add the mushrooms and spinach. Cook for an additional 4 minutes over medium heat.

4. Transfer the onion, spinach and mushroom mixture to a quiche pan sprayed with cooking spray. Spread evenly over the bottom.

5. Evenly distribute the shredded cheese over the onion, spinach, and mushroom mixture.

6. In a large bowl, combine flour and baking powder. Slowly whisk in the non-fat milk, then add the eggs, Dijon mustard, ½ teaspoon salt, and ½ teaspoon pepper. Whisk until well combined.

7. Pour the egg mixture over the onion, mushroom, spinach, and cheese layers in the quiche pan. Let sit at room temperature for 15-20 minutes.

8. Bake in the oven for 30-40 minutes, or until a toothpick inserted in the center comes out clean.

9. Let cool for 5 minutes before serving.

10. Enjoy!

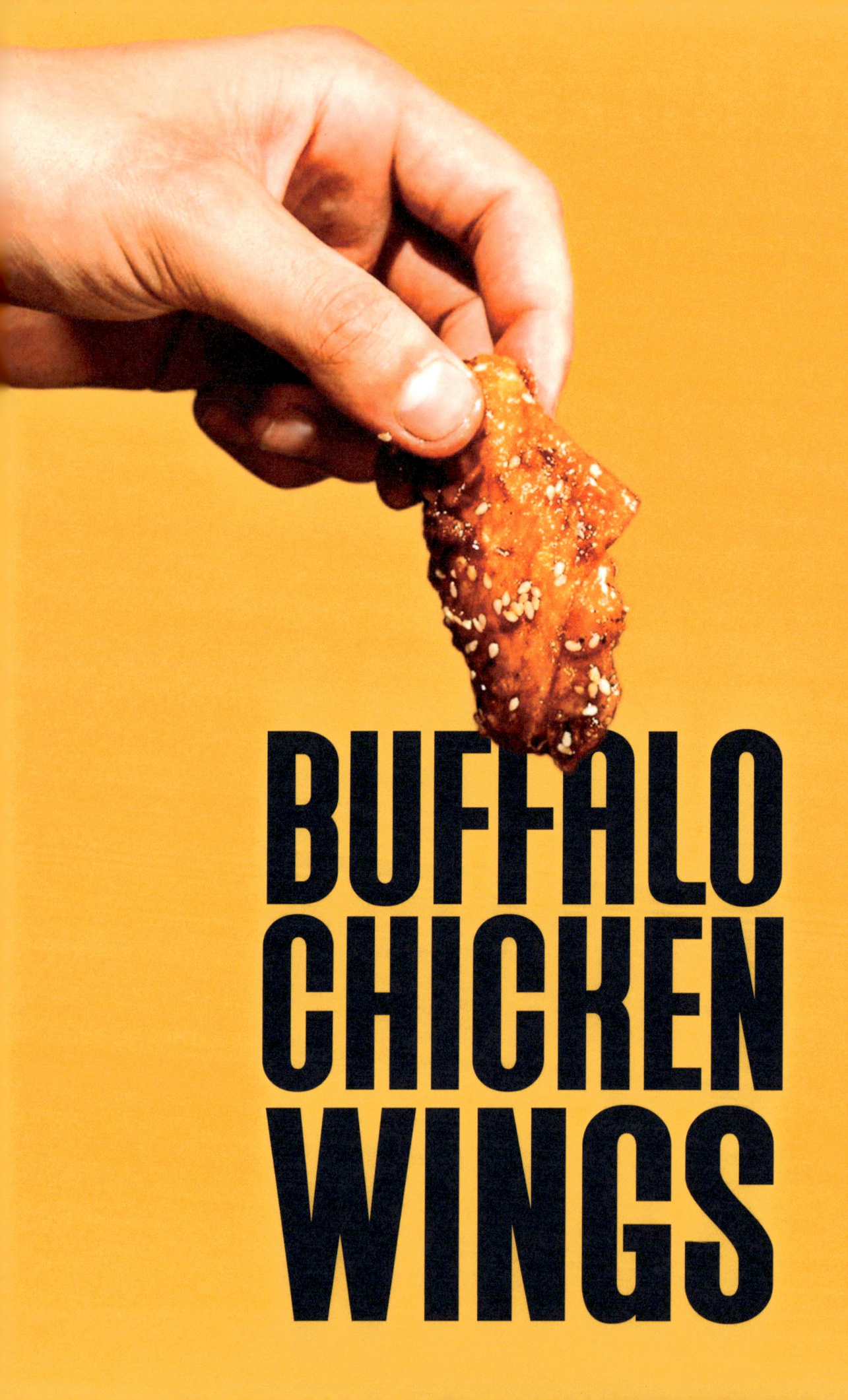

BUFFALO CHICKEN WINGS

BUFFALO CHICKEN WINGS

These spicy buffalo chicken wings are perfect for game day. Grab some friends and dig in!

INGREDIENTS

About 2 pounds of chicken wings

1 tablespoon buffalo sauce (for marinade)

½ tablespoon honey (for marinade)

1 tablespoon salt

½ tablespoon black pepper

½ tablespoon garlic powder

½ tablespoon onion powder

½ tablespoon smoked paprika

1 teaspoon baking powder

Dash of turmeric

Dash of oregano

Dash of thyme

2 tablespoons buffalo sauce (for sauce)

½ tablespoon honey (for sauce)

METHOD

1. Preheat oven to 400°F (200°C).

2. Pat chicken wings dry and place them in a bowl.

3. Add salt, honey, buffalo sauce, black pepper, garlic powder, onion powder, turmeric, smoked paprika, oregano, thyme, and baking powder to the bowl. Mix well to coat the wings. Marinate in the refrigerator overnight.

4. Arrange the chicken wings on a wire rack placed over a baking tray, ensuring they do not touch each other.

5. Bake for 30-40 minutes, or until the internal temperature reaches 165°F (75°C) and the wings are cooked through.

6. Remove the wings from the oven and place them in a bowl. Add the buffalo sauce and honey for the sauce, and mix well.

7. Enjoy!

Total Servings	3
Per Serving	
Calories	513.5
Added Sugar	4.2g
Fiber	1.6g
Fat	33.6g
Saturated Fat	9.3g
Protein	40.5g

Values are approximate and may vary based on ingredients used

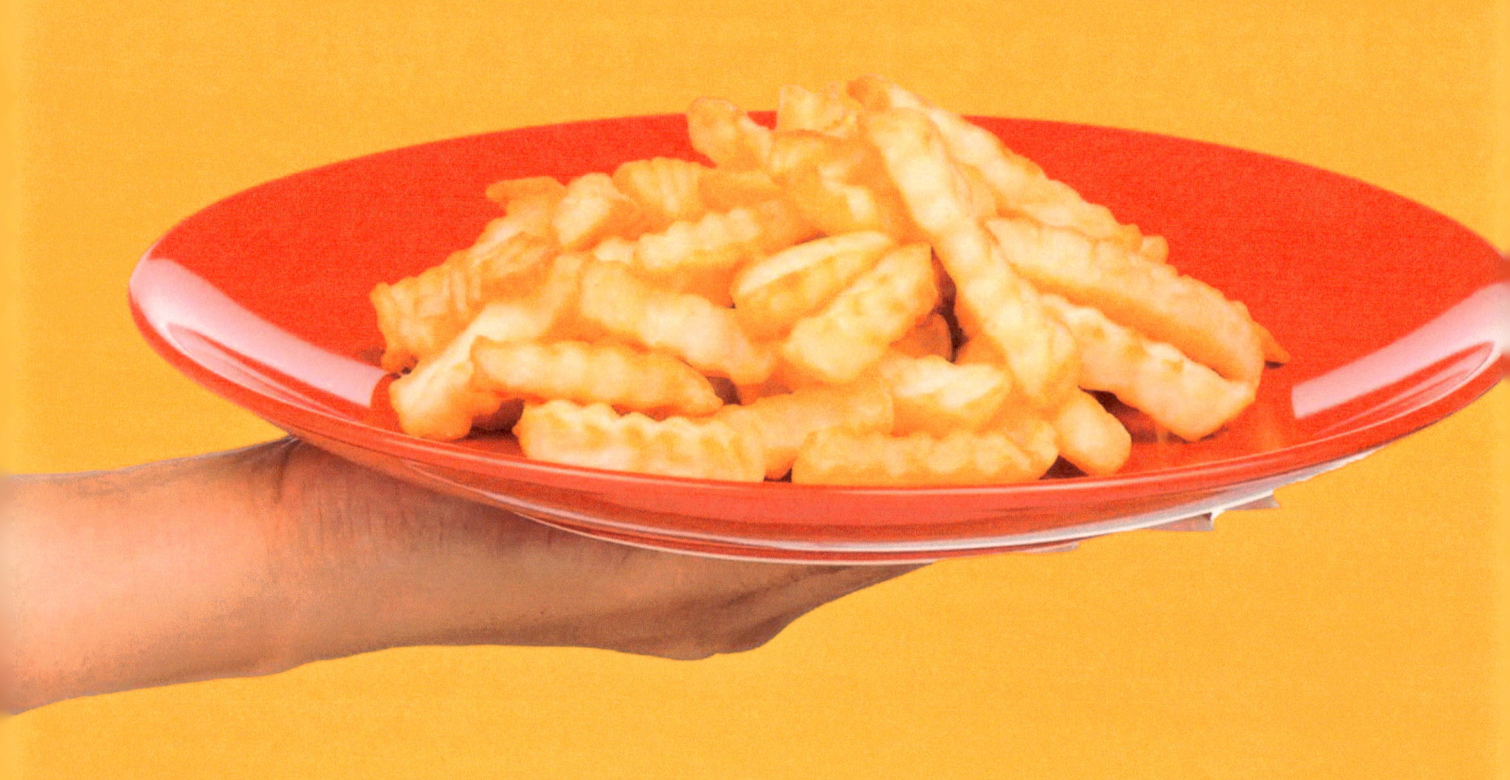

FRENCH FRIES

FRENCH FRIES

Homemade French fries that are crispy on the outside and soft on the inside. The ultimate comfort food.

INGREDIENTS

2 Yukon gold potatoes

1 teaspoon salt

½ teaspoon black pepper

½ teaspoon smoked paprika

½ teaspoon onion powder

½ teaspoon dried basil

½ teaspoon garlic powder

Dash of cayenne

Dash of oregano

Dash of turmeric

½ tablespoon olive oil

½ teaspoon baking powder

METHOD

1. Preheat oven to 300°F (150°C).

2. Peel the potatoes and slice them into your desired thickness for French fries. Soak the sliced potatoes in a bowl of cold water for 30 minutes to 1 hour.

3. Remove the potatoes from the water, pat them very dry, and place them in a dry bowl.

4. Add olive oil to the potatoes and mix to ensure each fry is coated with oil.

5. Season the fries with salt, black pepper, smoked paprika, onion powder, dried basil, garlic powder, cayenne, oregano, turmeric, and baking powder. Mix well to evenly coat the fries.

6. Arrange the fries on a wire rack placed over a baking tray, ensuring they do not touch each other.

7. Bake in the oven at 300°F for 20 minutes.

8. Increase the oven temperature to 425°F (220°C) and bake for an additional 10 minutes, or until the fries reach your desired crispiness.

9. Remove the fries from the oven and enjoy!

Total Servings	2
Per Serving	
Calories	194.5
Added Sugar	0g
Fiber	4.5g
Fat	3.8g
Saturated Fat	0.6g
Protein	4.0g

Values are approximate and may vary based on ingredients used

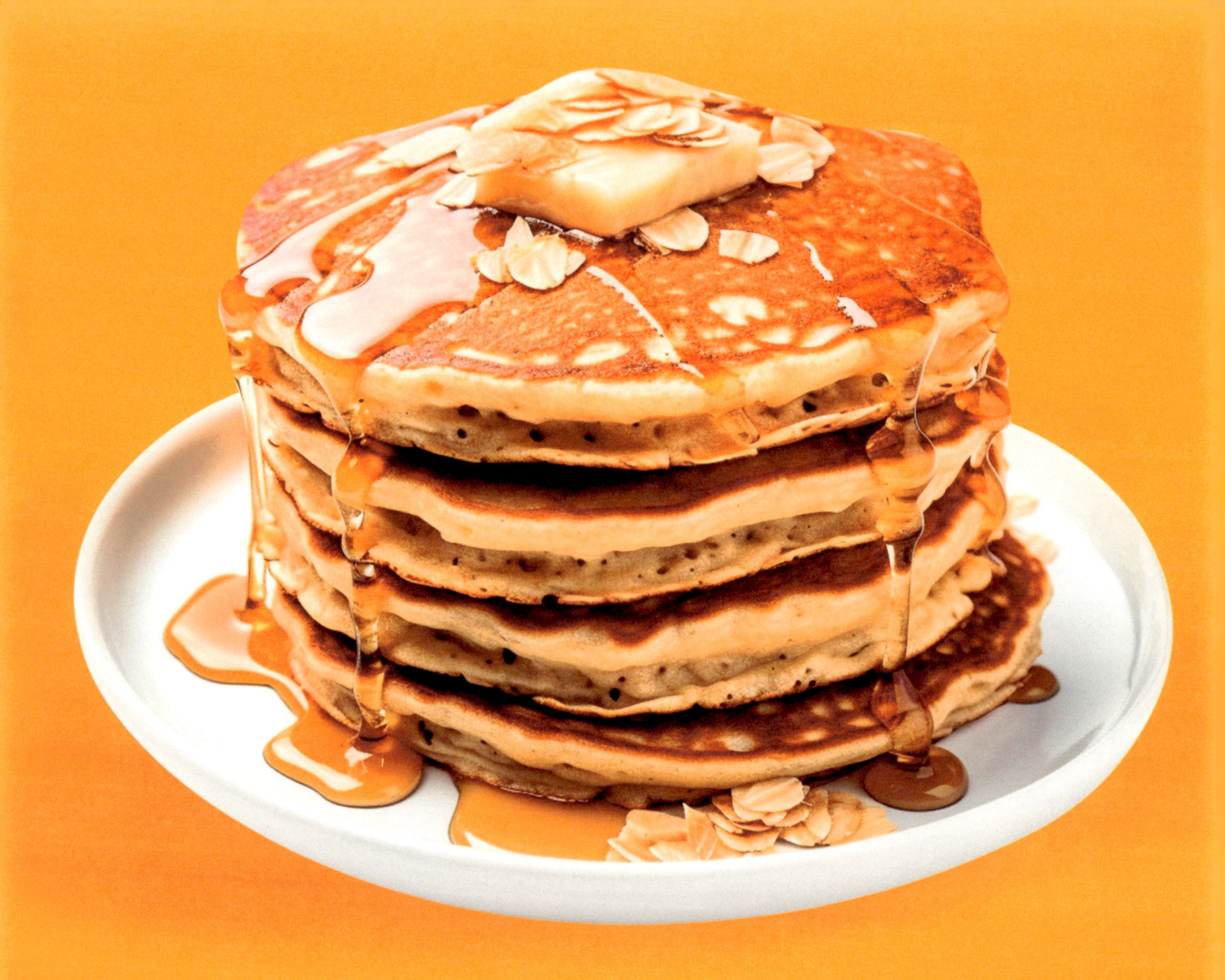

OATMEAL PANCAKES

OATMEAL PANCAKES

Start your day right with these hearty and healthy oatmeal pancakes. They're perfect for a filling breakfast.

INGREDIENTS

1 teaspoon melted and cooled coconut oil

2 tablespoons non-fat Greek yogurt

2 tablespoons non-fat milk

½ cup old-fashioned rolled oats

1 egg yolk

½ teaspoon baking powder

½ tablespoon maple syrup

Dash of vanilla extract

Dash of ground cinnamon

Pinch of salt

METHOD

1. Combine all ingredients except the rolled oats in a blender and blend until smooth.

2. Add the rolled oats to the blended mixture and let it sit for 10 minutes.

3. After 10 minutes, blend the mixture again until smooth but do not overblend.

4. Heat a non-stick pan over medium heat and spray with cooking spray.

5. Pour the batter onto the pan to form two medium-sized pancakes.

6. Cook until bubbles form on the top of the pancakes, then flip and cook for an additional 2 minutes.

7. Plate and serve.

8. Enjoy!

Total Servings	1
Per Serving	
Calories	299
Added Sugar	5.6g
Fiber	4.2g
Fat	12g
Saturated Fat	6.1g
Protein	11.1g

Values are approximate and may vary based on ingredients used

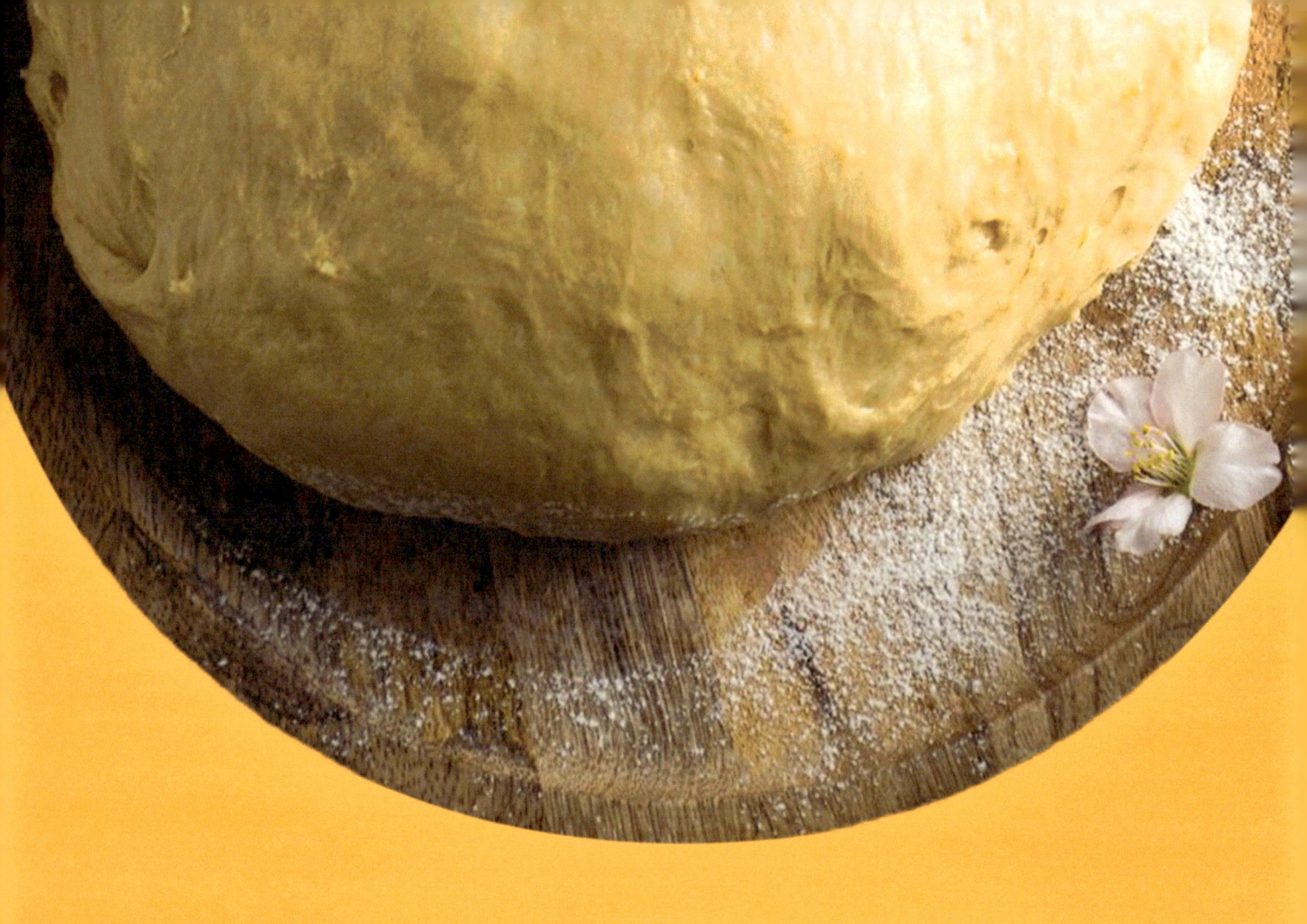

72 HOUR WHOLE WHEAT PIZZA DOUGH

WHOLE-WHEAT PIZZA

This 72-hour whole-wheat pizza dough is worth the wait. You'll never want store-bought again!

INGREDIENTS

FOR POOLISH:

150 grams (1 cup) 00 flour

150 ml water (about ⅔ cup)

2.5 grams (⅔ teaspoon) instant dry yeast

2.5 grams (1 teaspoon) honey

FOR DOUGH:

200 ml water (about ¾ cup)

100 grams (¾ cup) 00 flour

250 grams (2 cups) whole-wheat flour

13 grams (¾ tablespoon) salt

METHOD

1. In a large bowl, combine the water, yeast, and honey. Mix until combined.

2. Slowly add the flour, mixing until it forms a creamy paste. If the mixture is too doughy, add a bit more water.

3. Cover tightly and leave at room temperature for 2 hours, then refrigerate for 16-24 hours.

4. Remove the poolish from the fridge and let it sit at room temperature for 45 minutes with the cover still on.

5. In a larger bowl, mix the poolish with 200 ml (about ¾ cup) of water until well incorporated.

6. Add the salt and then gradually add both the 00 flour and whole-wheat flour, mixing until a dough forms. Use your hands to form the mixture into a dough ball. If too sticky, add more flour.

7. Knead the dough for 10 minutes, then cover and let it rest for 30 minutes.

8. Add olive oil to the dough and form it into a ball. Place the dough ball in a bowl, cover, and refrigerate for 24 hours.

9. After 24 hours, remove the dough from the fridge and divide it into 4 equal pieces.

10. Cover each piece in separate bowls and refrigerate for another 24 hours.

11. Your whole-wheat pizza dough is now ready to use for your pizza recipes throughout the book.

Total Servings	4 balls
Per Serving	
Calories	217.5
Added Sugar	0g
Fiber	4.4g
Fat	13.7g
Saturated Fat	2.9g
Protein	10.3g

Values are approximate and may vary based on ingredients used

NOTE: Using a cooking scale for this recipe is highly recommended for accuracy, as cup measurements can vary.

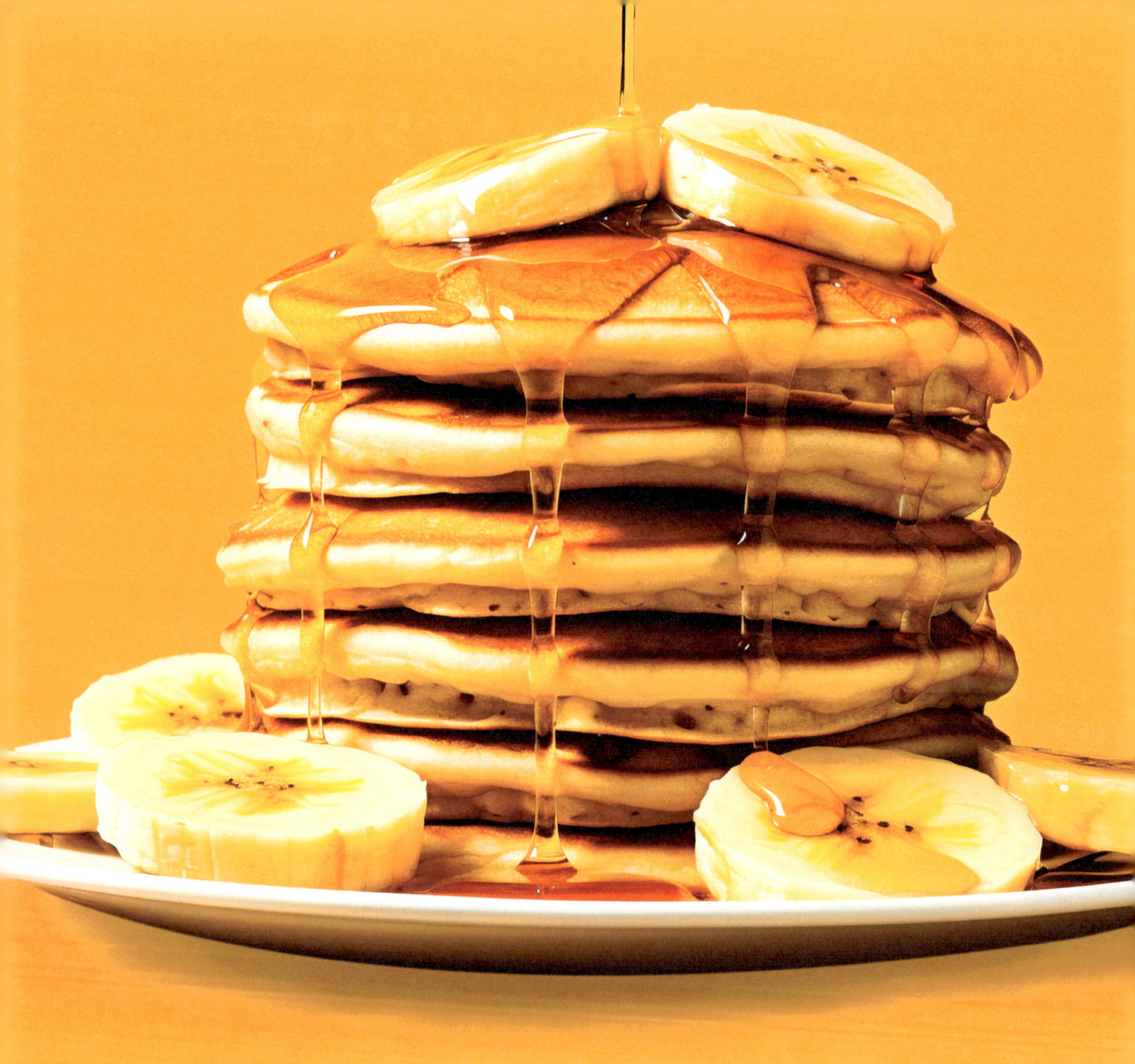

BANANA PANCAKES

BANANA PANCAKES

These banana pancakes are sweet, satisfying, and perfect for lazy weekend mornings.

INGREDIENTS

1 ripe banana

1 teaspoon melted and cooled coconut oil

2 tablespoons non-fat Greek yogurt

2 tablespoons non-fat milk

¾ cup old-fashioned rolled oats

1 egg yolk

½ teaspoon baking powder

½ tablespoon maple syrup

Dash of vanilla extract

Dash of ground cinnamon

Pinch of salt

METHOD

1. Combine all ingredients except the rolled oats in a blender and blend until smooth.

2. Add the rolled oats to the blended mixture and let it sit for 10 minutes.

3. After 10 minutes, blend the mixture again until smooth but do not overblend.

4. Heat a non-stick pan over medium heat and spray with cooking spray.

5. Pour the batter onto the pan to form two medium-sized pancakes.

6. Cook until bubbles form on the top of the pancakes, then flip and cook for an additional 2 minutes.

7. Plate and serve.

8. Enjoy!

Total Servings	2
Per Serving	
Calories	**239.5**
Added Sugar	**2.8g**
Fiber	**4.6g**
Fat	**7g**
Saturated Fat	**3.2g**
Protein	**7.4g**

Values are approximate and may vary based on ingredients used

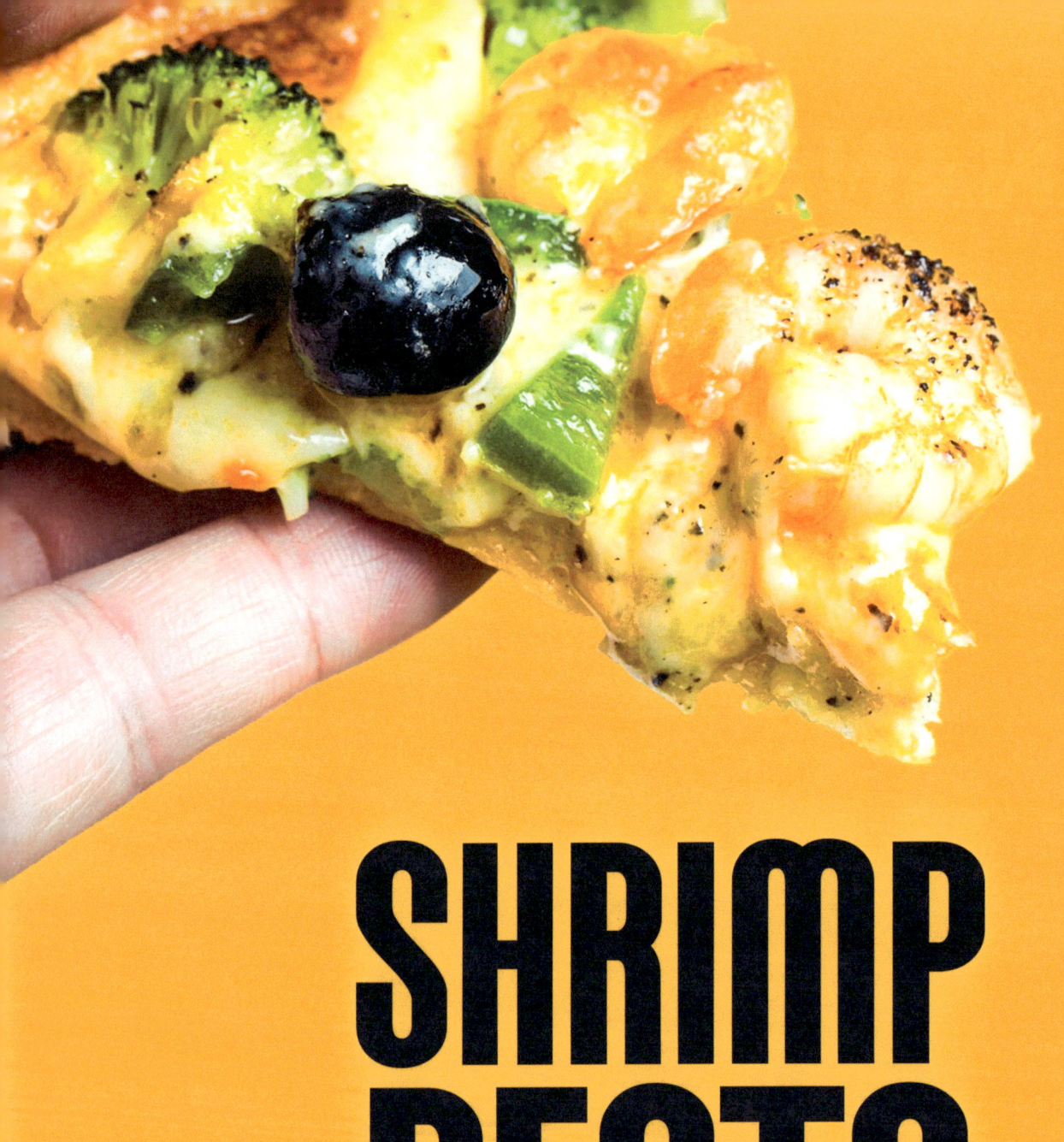

SHRIMP PESTO PIZZA

SHRIMP PESTO PIZZA

Take pizza night to the next level with this delicious shrimp pesto pizza. Gourmet vibes at home!

INGREDIENTS

1 ball of whole-wheat pizza dough (recipe in this book)

5 raw shrimp, deveined and tail off

2 tablespoons of pesto (recipe in this book)

2 tablespoons of fresh mozzarella

2 tablespoons of pizza sauce (recipe in this book)

¼ teaspoon garlic powder

½ teaspoon salt

¼ teaspoon pepper

¼ teaspoon turmeric

Pizza stone

Pizza peel

METHOD

1. Place your pizza stone in the oven and preheat it to the highest temperature possible. The pizza stone should be in the oven for at least an hour before putting the pizza in.

2. Season the raw, deveined, and detailed shrimp with salt, garlic powder, pepper, and turmeric.

3. Stretch out the pizza dough into a 12-inch round. Instructions for dough preparation can be found in this book. Ensure to flour both sides of the dough generously to prevent sticking.

4. Once the dough is formed, move it onto the pizza peel. Quickly and evenly spread the pizza sauce over the top of the dough, leaving the crust uncovered. Slide the pizza onto the preheated pizza stone.

5. Cook on the pizza stone for a few minutes (the time will vary depending on the heat of your oven) until the sauce begins to dry out slightly and the crust puffs up.

6. Remove the pizza from the oven using the pizza peel. Scatter the seasoned shrimp evenly around the pizza. Drizzle the pesto over the pizza and scatter the mozzarella evenly over the pizza.

7. Return the pizza to the oven and cook until the cheese is crispy.

8. Remove the pizza from the oven, slice, and enjoy!

Total Servings	2
Per Serving	
Calories	330
Added Sugar	0g
Fiber	5.7g
Fat	12.4g
Saturated Fat	2.8g
Protein	13.4g

Values are approximate and may vary based on ingredients used

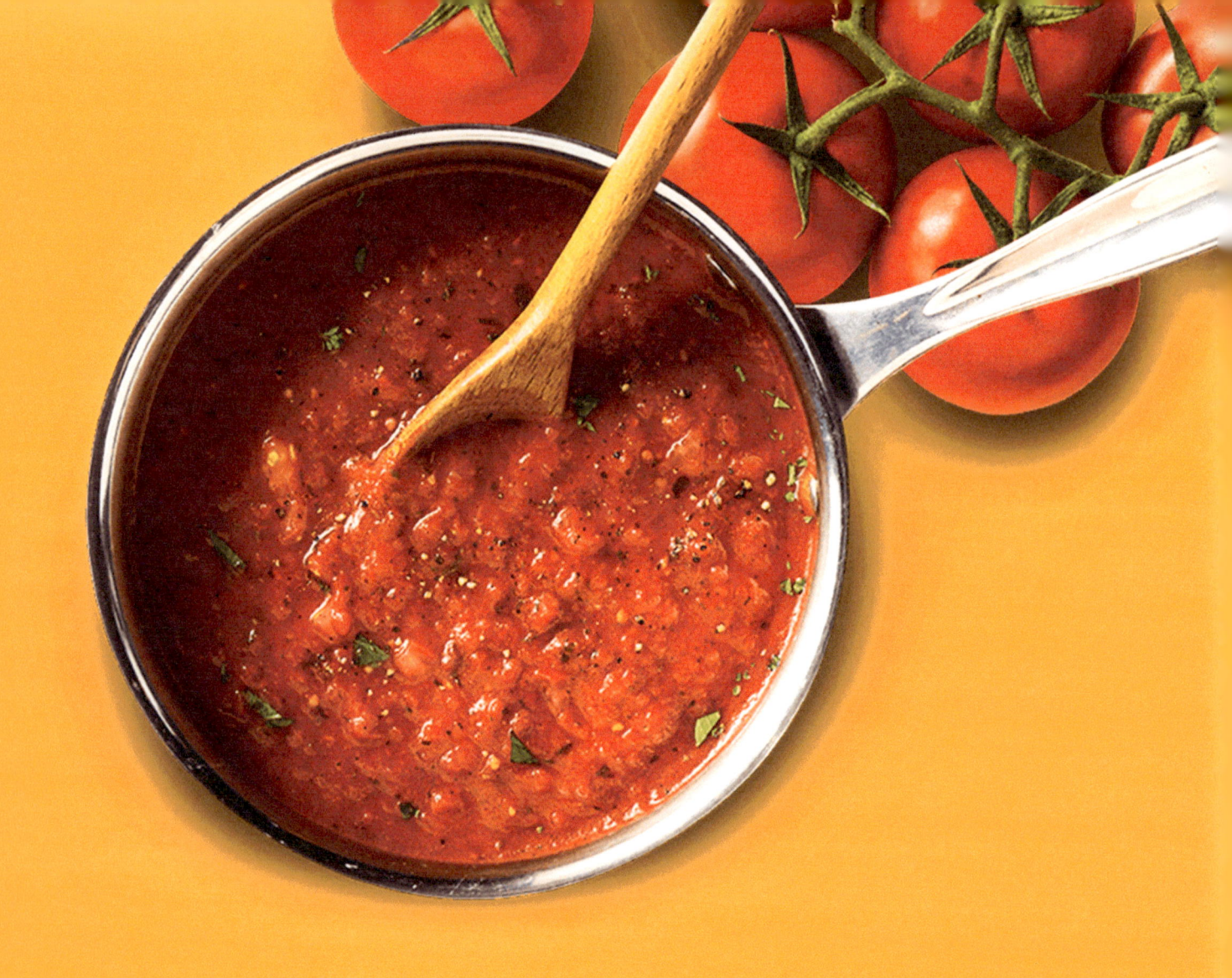

PIZZA SAUCE

PIZZA SAUCE

Homemade pizza sauce is a game-changer. It's simple, tasty, and perfect for all your pizza creations.

INGREDIENTS

1 28 oz can whole peeled tomatoes (recommended brands: Alta Cucina and Bianco Dinapoli)

1 teaspoon salt

1 teaspoon dried oregano

½ teaspoon dried basil

METHOD

1. Using an immersion blender, combine all ingredients.
2. Blend until very smooth.
3. Store in the refrigerator.

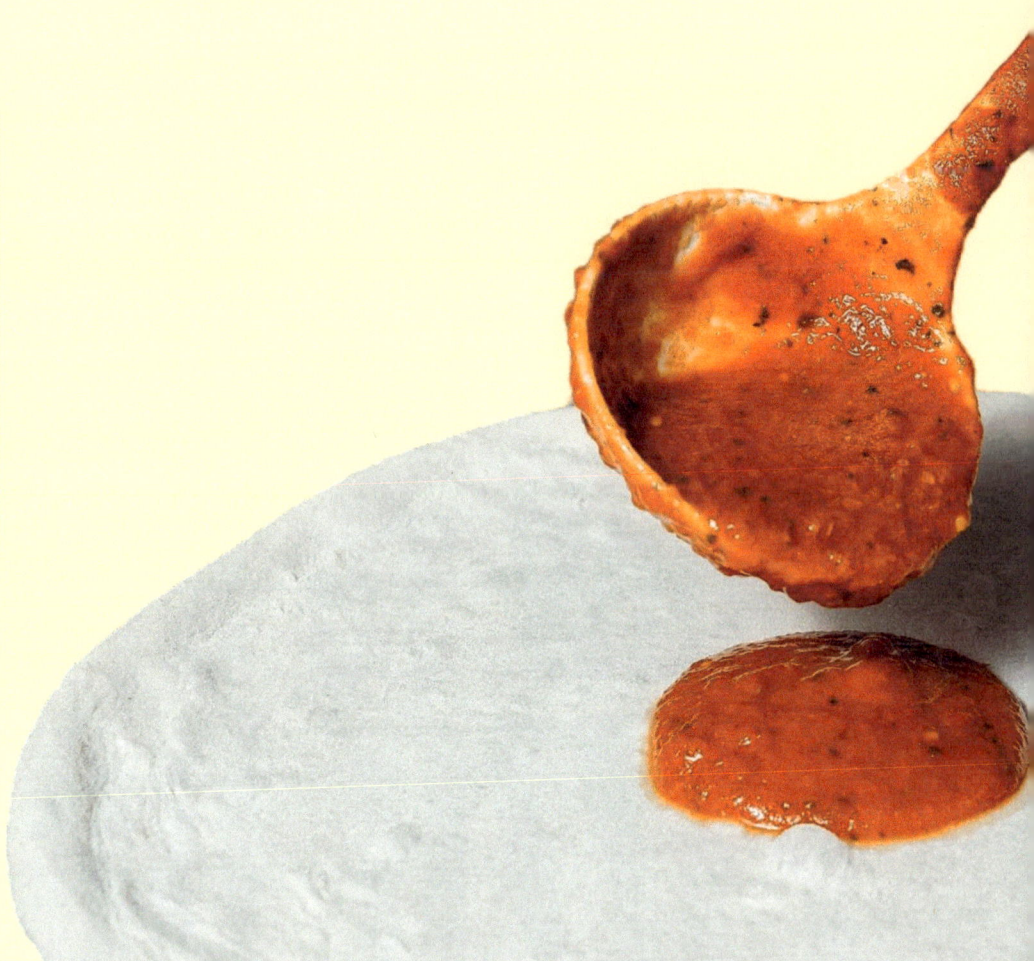

Total Servings	7
Per Serving	
Calories	19.1
Added Sugar	0g
Fiber	1.6g
Fat	0.1g
Saturated Fat	0.0g
Protein	0.9g

Values are approximate and may vary based on ingredients used

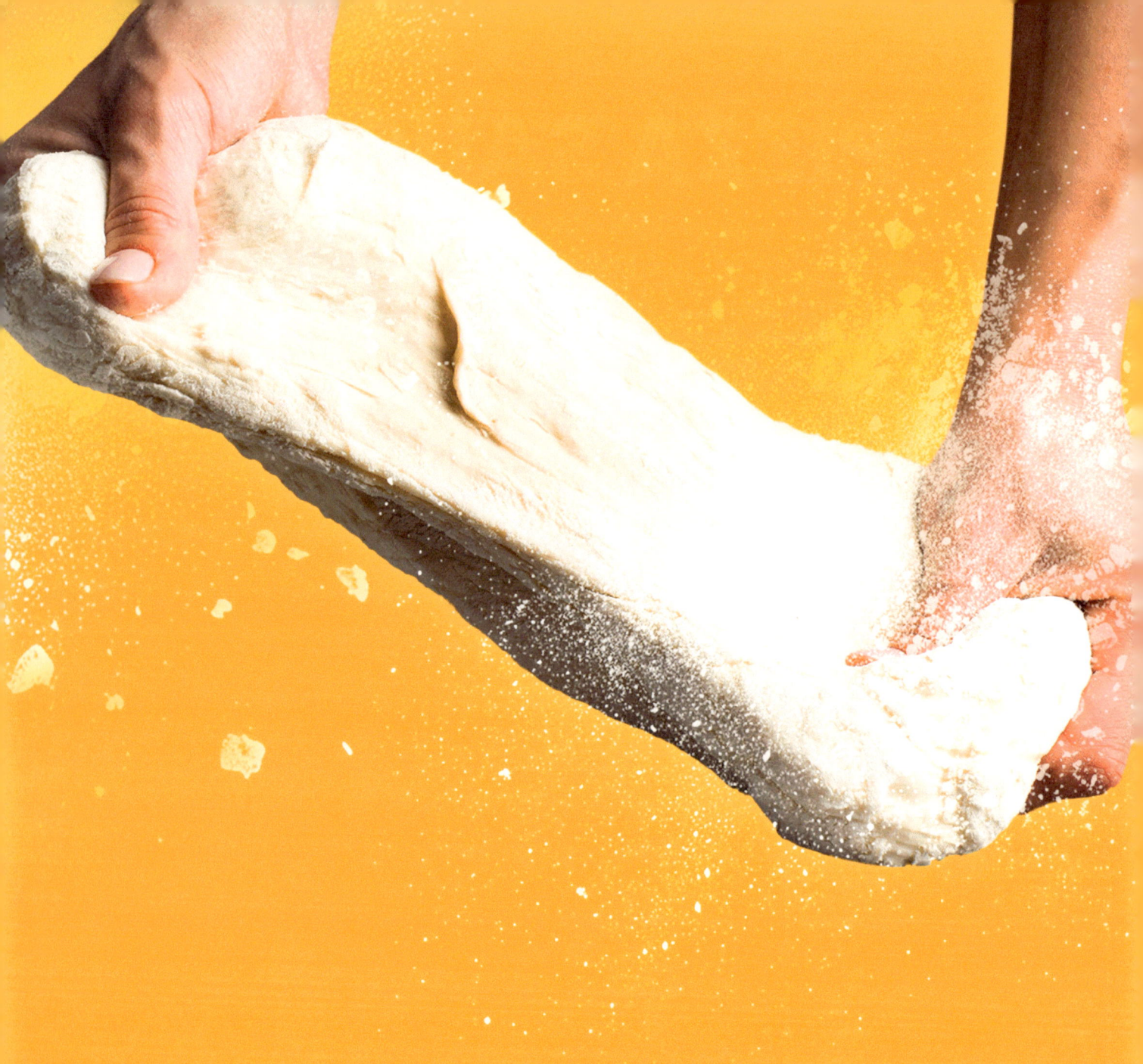

HOW TO STRETCH PIZZA DOUGH

HOW TO STRETCH PIZZA DOUGH

Mastering pizza dough stretching is a must. Your homemade pizzas will thank you!

INGREDIENTS

1 ball of pizza dough

METHOD

1. Place the ball of pizza dough on a well-floured surface to prevent sticking.

2. Gently press the dough with your fingertips, starting from the center and working outwards, to flatten it into a disk about 6 inches in diameter.

3. Pick up the dough, holding it with both hands at the edges, and let gravity help stretch it as you rotate the dough in a circular motion.

4. Place the dough over your knuckles, carefully stretching it by rotating and pulling your hands apart slightly to widen the circle. Ensure you maintain an even thickness.

5. If the dough becomes too resistant or starts to tear, let it rest on the floured surface for 5-10 minutes to relax the gluten before continuing.

6. Continue stretching until the dough is about 12 inches in diameter and uniformly thin, with a slightly thicker edge for the crust.

7. Transfer the stretched dough to a well-floured pizza peel, ensuring it can slide easily before adding toppings and baking.

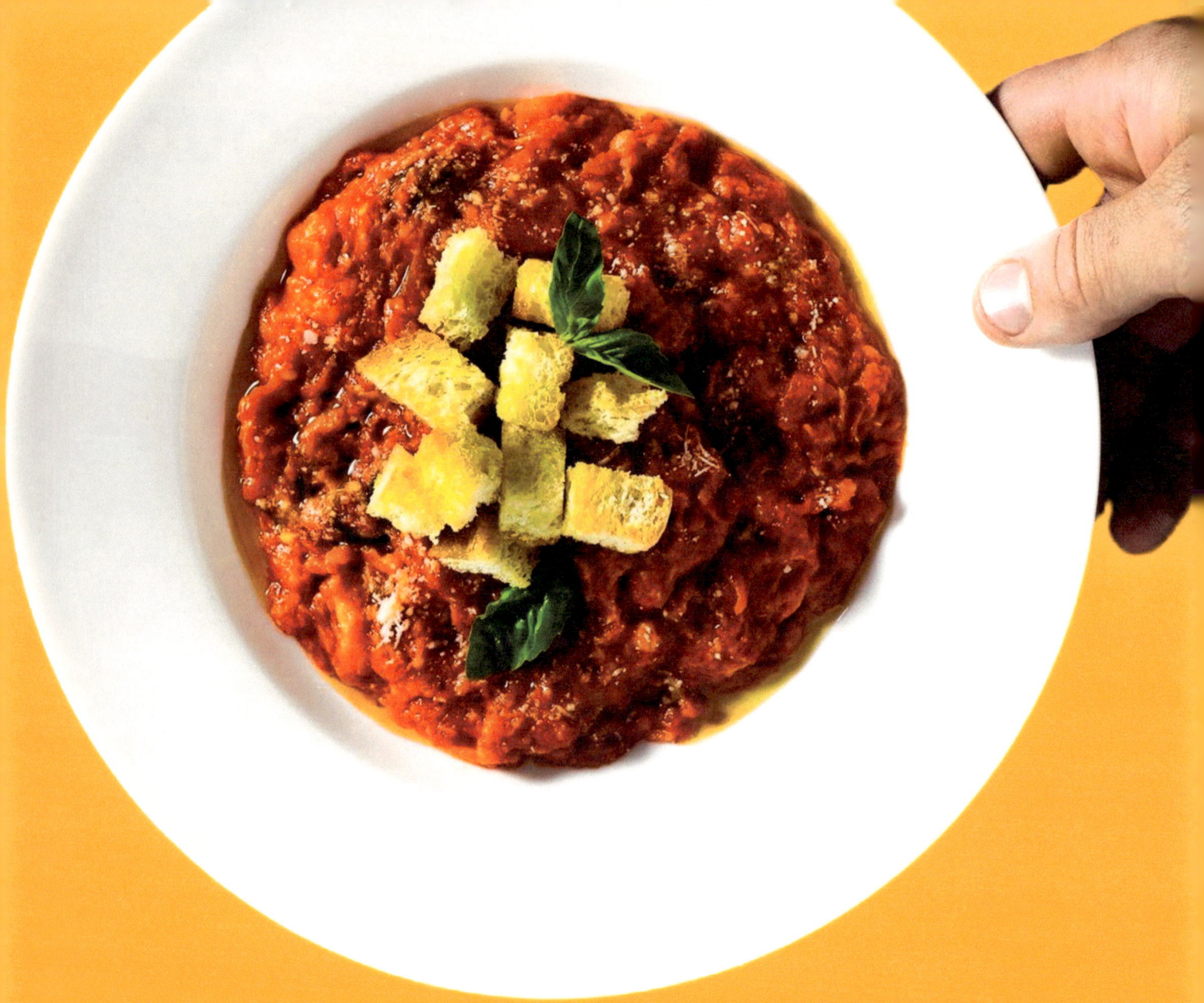

PAPPA AL POMODORO

PAPPA AL POMODORO

Warm up with this comforting Italian tomato and bread soup. It's like a hug in a bowl.

INGREDIENTS

1 28 oz can of whole peeled tomatoes

7 slices of stale sourdough bread

About 10 fresh basil leaves

2 teaspoons extra virgin olive oil

1 and ⅔ cups vegetable stock

4 cloves garlic, minced

½ yellow onion, diced

Salt and pepper to taste

METHOD

1. If you do not have stale bread, place the slices in the oven with the fan on at 300°F. Toast until the pieces are hard but not brown, about 15 minutes, flipping halfway through.

2. Add olive oil to a large saucepan and heat over medium. Add diced onions with a pinch of salt and stir. Cook until the onions barely start to brown, about 7 minutes.

3. While the onions are cooking, pour the can of tomatoes into a large bowl. Using your hands, crush the tomatoes until there are a few small chunks remaining.

4. Once the onions are done, add minced garlic to the pot and cook for an additional 30 seconds, stirring constantly.

5. Add the crushed tomatoes from the bowl to the saucepan along with about 5 basil leaves. Cook for 1 minute, stirring constantly.

6. Add half of the vegetable stock to the saucepan and cook for 7 minutes, stirring occasionally.

7. Add the remaining vegetable stock and cook for another 3 minutes.

8. Tear the stale bread into bite sized pieces and add it to the saucepan, stirring constantly. Adjust the heat to low and cook until the bread is mushy.

9. Once the bread is mushy, season with salt and pepper to taste. Add the other 5 basil leaves

10. Serve and enjoy.

Total Servings	4
Per Serving	
Calories	222.5
Added Sugar	0g
Fiber	4.5g
Fat	3.2g
Saturated Fat	0.5g
Protein	7.4g

Values are approximate and may vary based on ingredients used

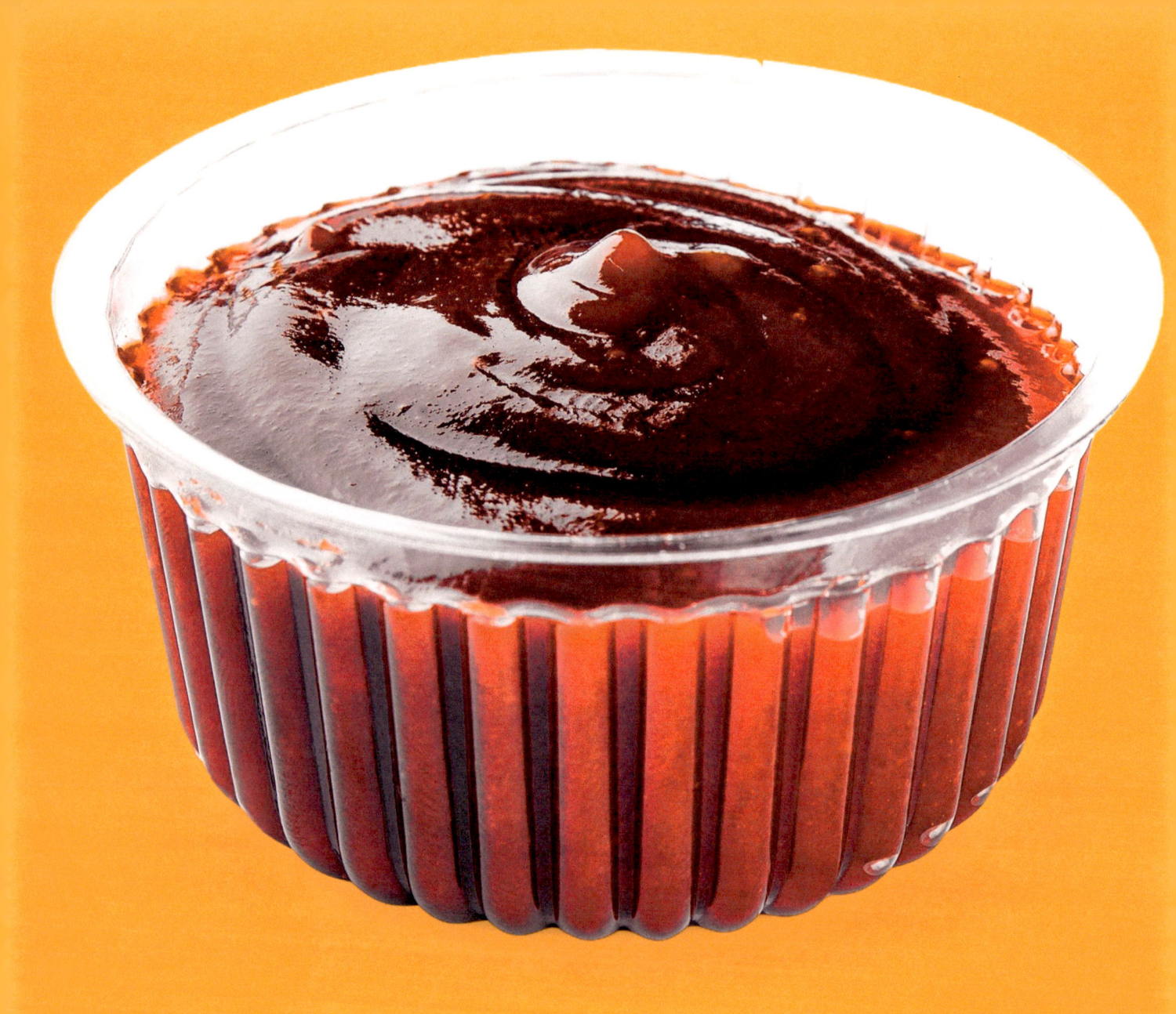

BARBECUE SAUCE

BARBECUE SAUCE

Whip up this tangy, sweet barbecue sauce for all your grilling needs. Perfect on ribs, burgers, and more!

INGREDIENTS

½ yellow onion, diced

1 teaspoon extra virgin olive oil

1 clove garlic, minced

½ cup tomato sauce

¼ cup water

2 tablespoons maple syrup

1 tablespoon apple cider vinegar

½ tablespoon balsamic vinegar

1 teaspoon soy sauce

½ tablespoon molasses

½ teaspoon smoked paprika

Dash of chili powder

½ teaspoon salt

Dash of black pepper

Total Servings	8
Per Serving	
Calories	22.8
Added Sugar	2.4g
Fiber	0.3g
Fat	0.6g
Saturated Fat	0.1g
Protein	0.3g
Sodium	226g

Values are approximate and may vary based on ingredients used

METHOD

1. Add extra virgin olive oil to a pot on medium heat.

2. Once hot, add the diced onion with a pinch of salt. Stir occasionally and cook for about 8 minutes, or until the onions start to caramelize.

3. Add minced garlic to the pot and cook for 1 minute.

4. Add water to the pot to deglaze and cook for 1 minute.

5. Add tomato sauce, maple syrup, apple cider vinegar, balsamic vinegar, soy sauce, molasses, smoked paprika, chili powder, salt, and black pepper.

6. Stir until all ingredients are combined and bring the pot to a simmer.

7. Let it simmer for 5 minutes.

8. After 5 minutes, remove the pot from heat and let it cool for 20 minutes.

9. Transfer the mixture to a blender and blend until very smooth.

10. Your barbecue sauce is now ready. Enjoy!

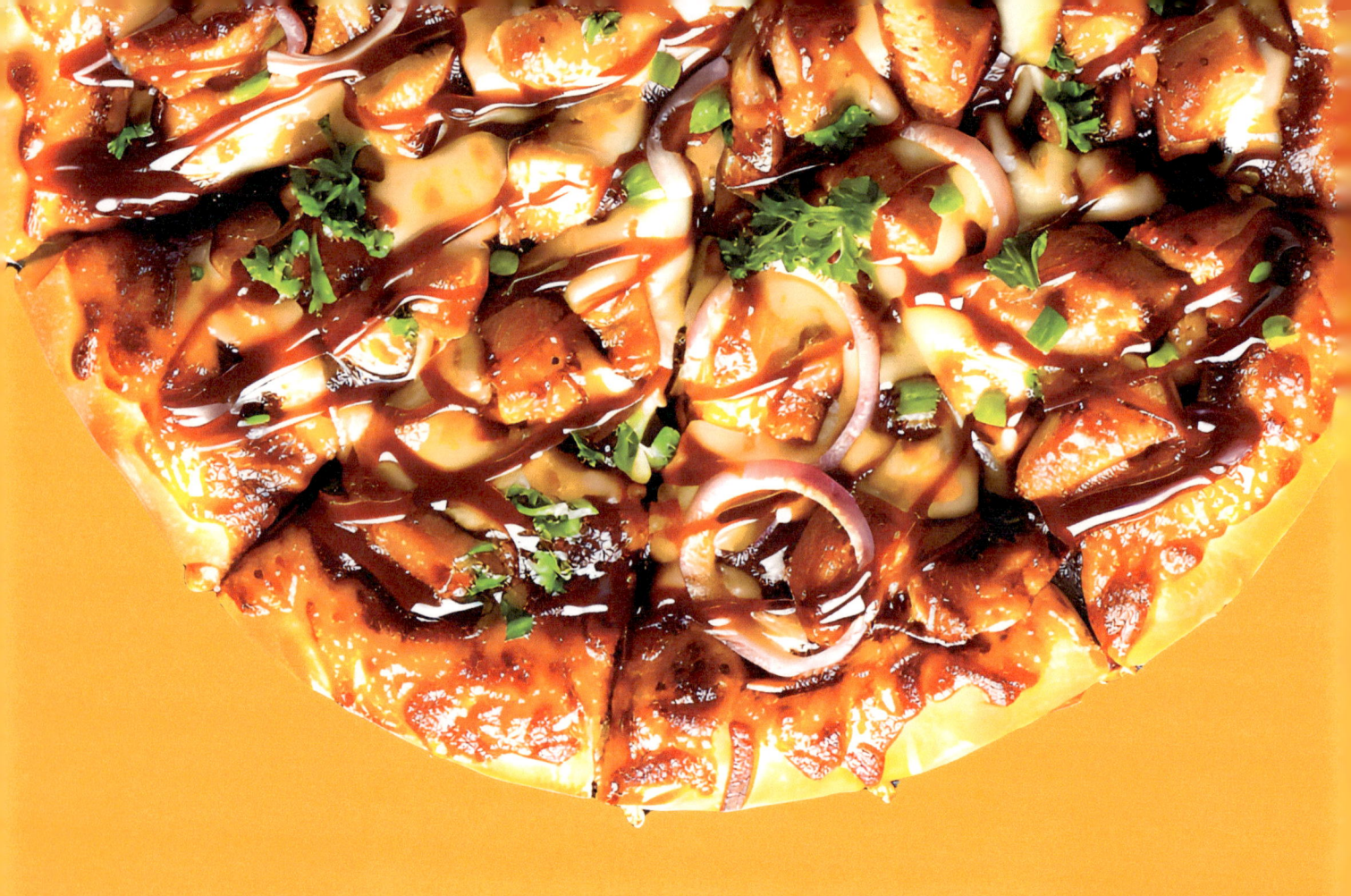

BARBECUE CHICKEN PIZZA

BARBECUE CHICKEN PIZZA

Combine BBQ and pizza for a match made in heaven. This barbecue chicken pizza is a total win.

INGREDIENTS

1 whole-wheat pizza ball

3 chicken thighs, cut into cubes

1 tablespoon smoked paprika

1 teaspoon turmeric

1 tablespoon salt

1 teaspoon olive oil

1 tablespoon black pepper

1 tablespoon garlic powder

3 tablespoons barbecue sauce (recipe in this book)

2 cups water

2 tablespoons fresh mozzarella

½ cup chicken stock

Pizza stone

Pizza peel

Total Servings	2
Per Serving	
Calories	514.9
Added Sugar	4.5g
Fiber	9.3g
Fat	22.3g
Saturated Fat	5.9g
Protein	28.6g

Values are approximate and may vary based on ingredients used

METHOD

1. Put the pizza stone in the oven and preheat it to the highest temperature possible.

2. Season the chicken thighs with smoked paprika, turmeric, salt, black pepper, and garlic powder.

3. Add olive oil to a pot and set the heat to medium. Once hot, add the seasoned chicken and cook until browned on all sides.

4. Add water and chicken stock to the pot. Bring to a boil and cook for 20 minutes.

5. Remove the chicken from the pot and shred it.

6. Add 2 tablespoons of barbecue sauce to the shredded chicken and stir to combine.

7. Stretch out the pizza dough into a 12-inch round. Instructions for dough preparation can be found in this book. Be sure to flour both sides of the dough generously to prevent sticking.

8. Once the dough is formed, move it onto the pizza peel. Quickly and evenly spread 2 tablespoons of barbecue sauce over the top of the dough, leaving the crust uncovered. Slide the pizza onto the preheated pizza stone.

9. Cook on the pizza stone for a few minutes (the time will vary depending on the heat of your oven) until the sauce begins to dry out slightly and the crust puffs up.

10. Remove the pizza from the oven using the pizza peel. Scatter the shredded chicken evenly around the pizza. Scatter the mozzarella evenly over the pizza.

11. Return the pizza to the oven and cook until the cheese is crispy.

12. Remove the pizza from the oven, slice, and enjoy!

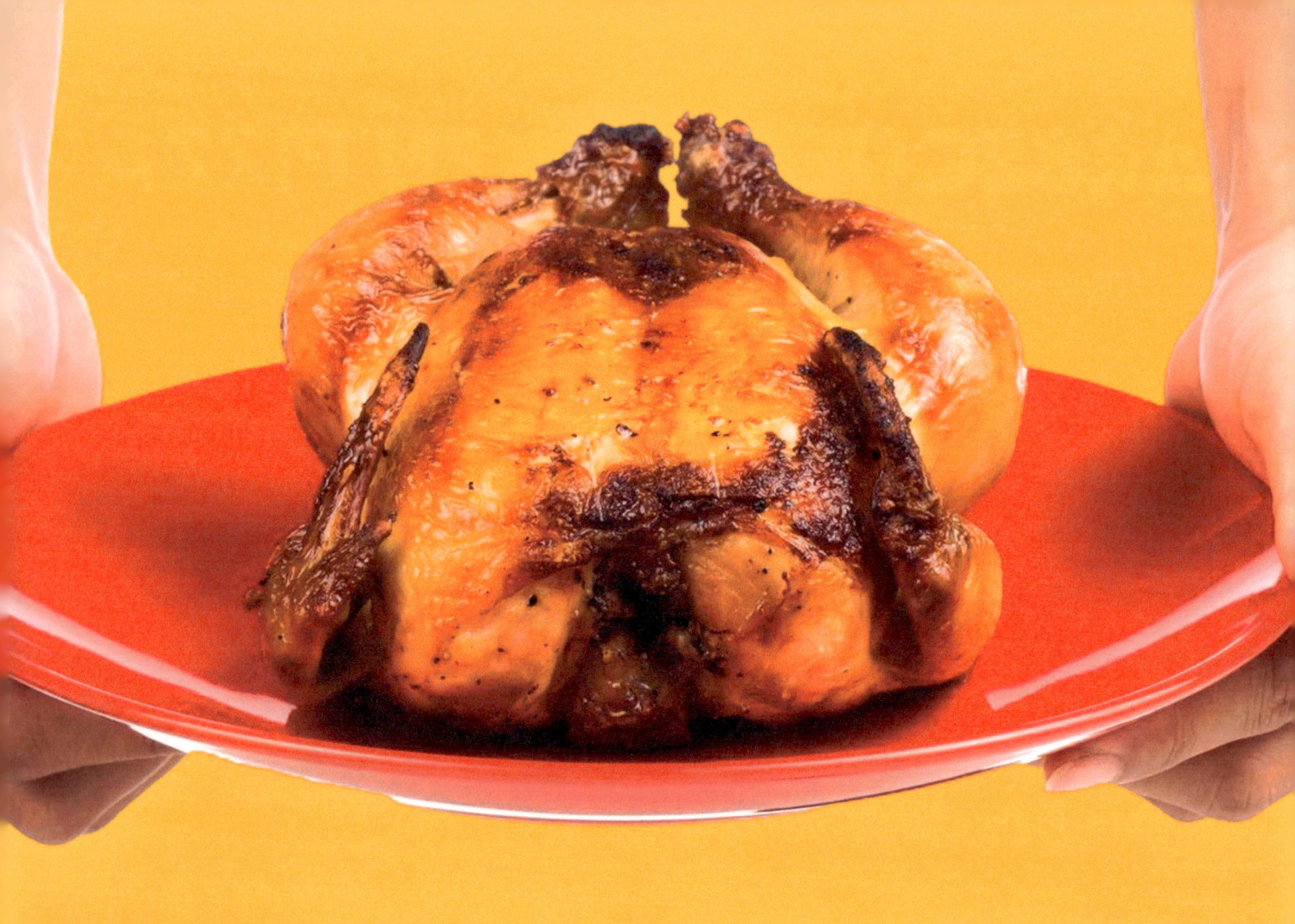

THE BEST ROASTED CHICKEN

THE BEST ROASTED CHICKEN

This roasted chicken is juicy, flavorful, and sure to impress. A perfect go-to dinner.

INGREDIENTS

1 whole raw chicken

2 tablespoons avocado oil

2 tablespoons salt

1 tablespoon black pepper

1 tablespoon garlic powder

1 lemon, chopped into 4 pieces

Butcher's twine

METHOD

1. Preheat the oven to 300°F.

2. Pat down the whole raw chicken and remove the guts from the cavity. Pat everything dry again.

3. Rub the entire chicken with avocado oil. Season every part of the chicken, including the inner cavity, with salt, black pepper, and garlic powder.

4. Place the lemon pieces inside the inner cavity of the chicken.

5. Using butcher's twine, tie the two legs to the neck.

6. Place the chicken on a wire rack if you have one, or if you don't, you can place it directly on a baking tray.

7. Cook the chicken in the oven for 2-3 hours, or until the internal temperature reaches 165°F.

8. Remove the chicken from the oven and let it rest for 20 minutes.

9. Enjoy!

Total Servings	5
Per Serving	
Calories	493
Added Sugar	0g
Fiber	1.6g
Fat	38.9g
Saturated Fat	10.3g
Protein	34.6g

Values are approximate and may vary based on ingredients used

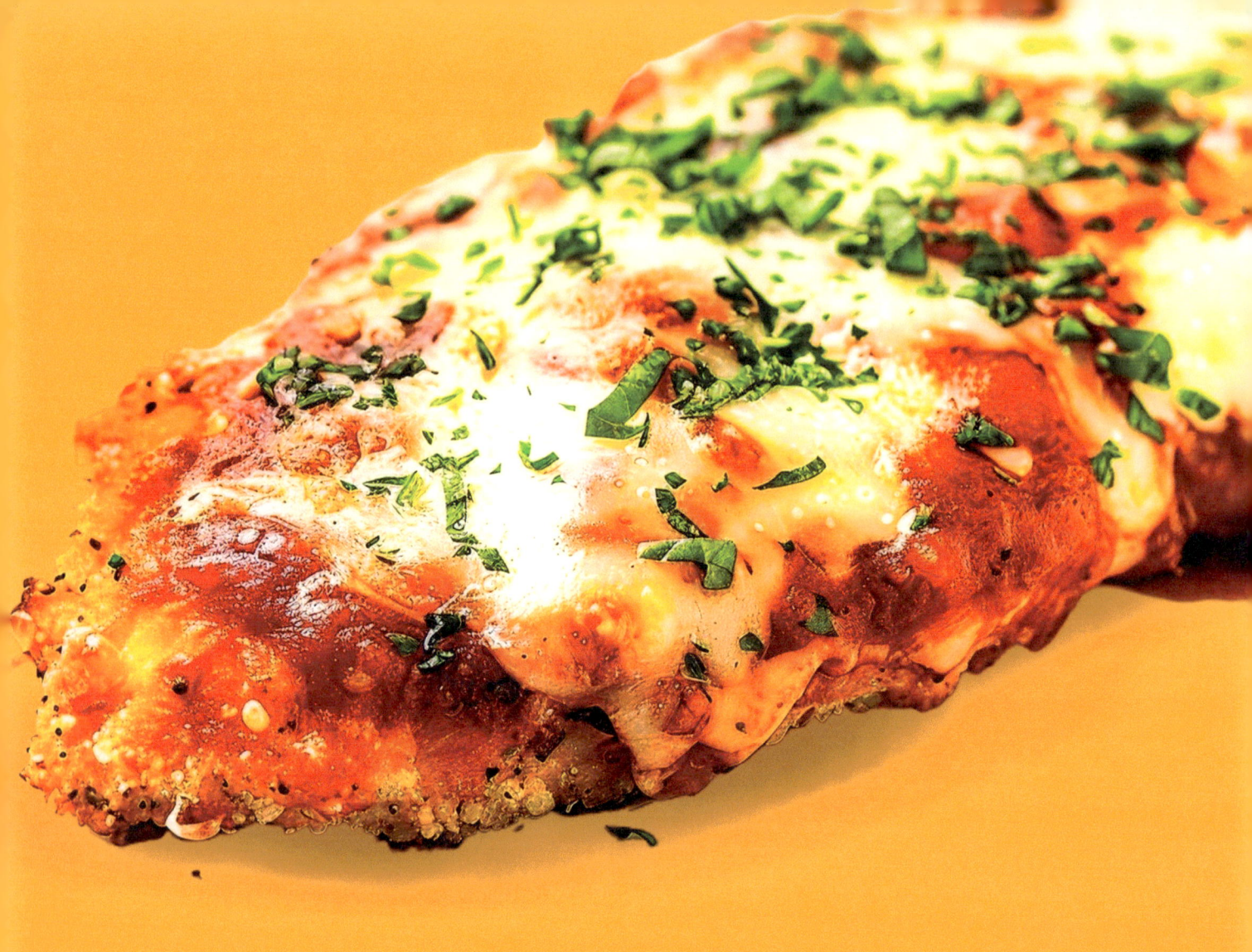

CHICKEN PARMESAN

CHICKEN PARMESAN

Classic chicken Parmesan that's crispy, cheesy, and absolutely delicious. A true comfort food favorite.

INGREDIENTS

1 chicken breast, pounded thin

½ cup pizza sauce (recipe in this book)

3-4 slices of fresh mozzarella cheese

¼ cup finely crushed cornflakes

¼ cup whole-wheat flour

2 egg whites

1 teaspoon salt

1 teaspoon smoked paprika

1 teaspoon garlic powder

1 teaspoon black pepper

METHOD

1. Prepare three separate bowls: one with whole-wheat flour, one with crushed cornflakes, and one with egg whites.

2. Season the whole-wheat flour with salt, smoked paprika, garlic powder, and black pepper. Stir to combine.

3. Coat the chicken breast with the seasoned whole-wheat flour, then dip it in the egg whites, and finally coat it completely with the crushed cornflakes.

4. Spray all sides of the coated chicken with cooking spray and place it in the air fryer at 400°F for 7 minutes.

5. Flip the chicken and cook at 400°F for an additional 5 minutes.

6. Pour the pizza sauce over the chicken breast and place the slices of mozzarella on top. Cook for an additional 3-4 minutes at 400°F, or until the cheese is melted.

7. Ensure the internal temperature of the chicken is at least 165°F.

8. Enjoy!

Total Servings	1
Per Serving	
Calories	489.9
Added Sugar	1g
Fiber	7.2g
Fat	11.3g
Saturated Fat	5.1g
Protein	51.2g

Values are approximate and may vary based on ingredients used

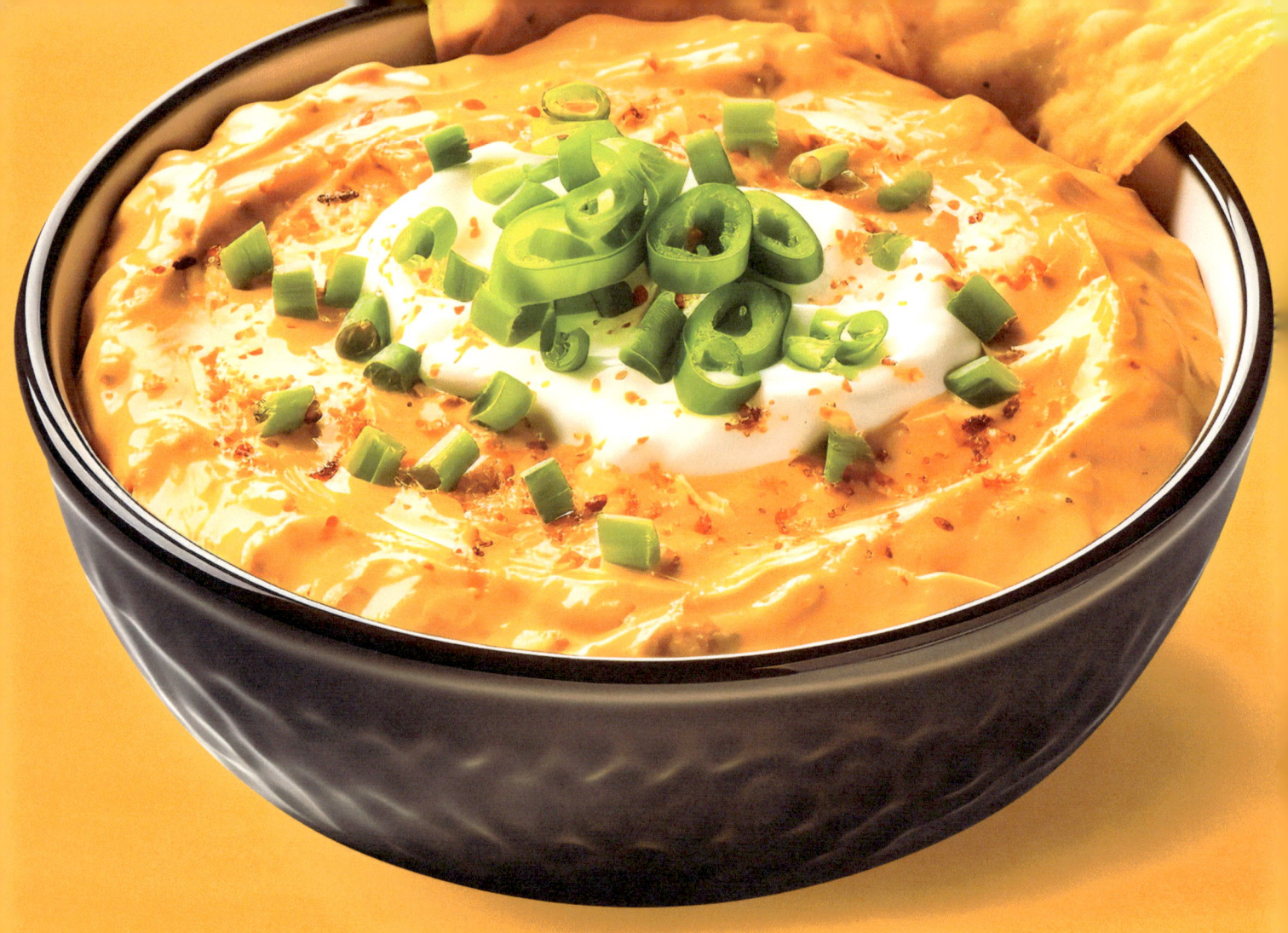

BUFFALO RANCH SAUCE

BUFFALO RANCH SAUCE

This buffalo ranch sauce is a spicy, zesty addition to any dish. Perfect for dipping, drizzling, and more.

8 SERVINGS

INGREDIENTS

1 cup Frank's Red Hot sauce

½ cup light ranch (recipe in this book)

1 teaspoon honey

METHOD

1. Combine all ingredients in a squeeze bottle.
2. Shake well to mix thoroughly.
3. Enjoy!

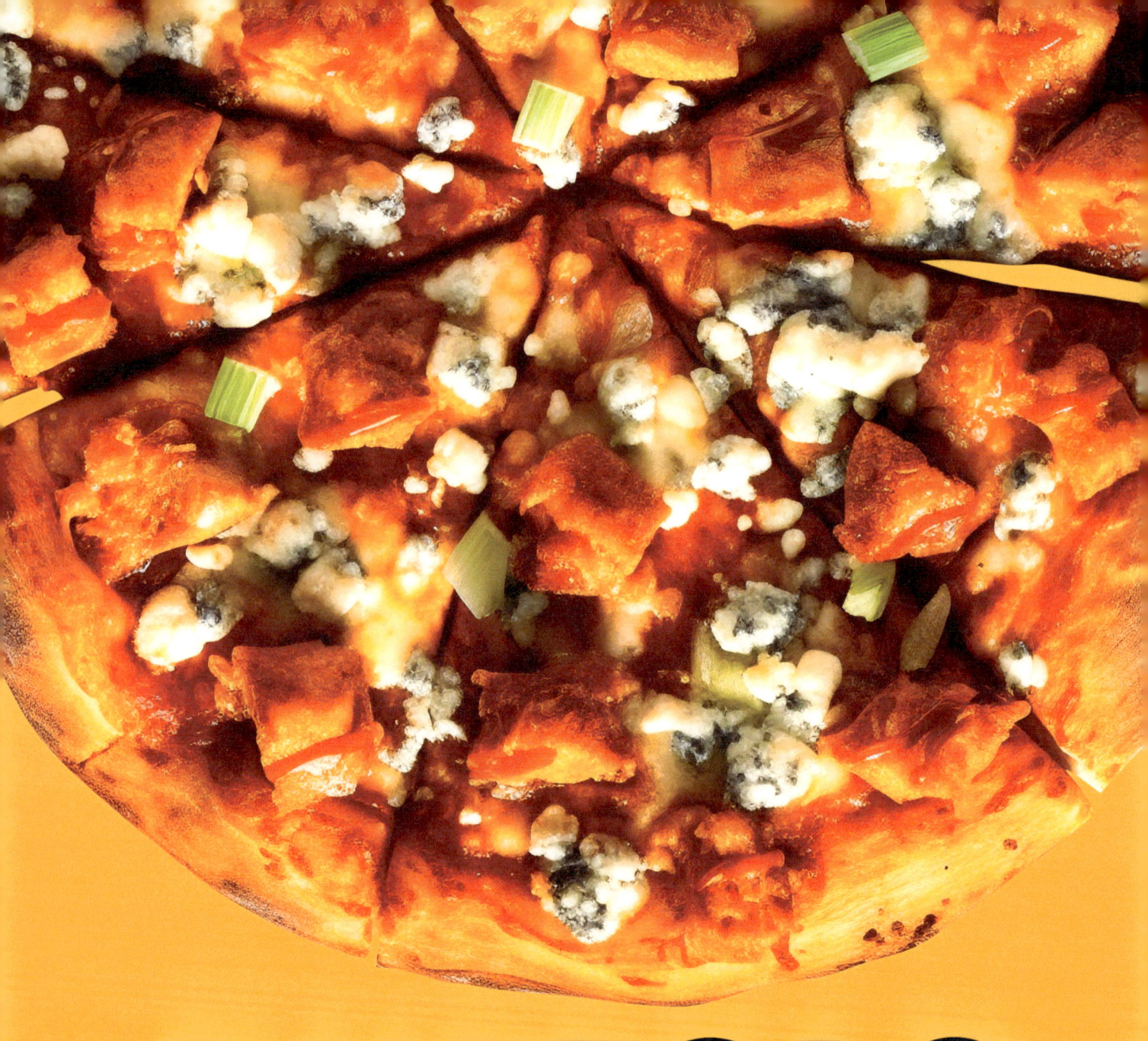

BUFFALO CHICKEN PIZZA

BUFFALO CHICKEN PIZZA

Spicy buffalo chicken pizza is here to take your pizza game to the next level. It's epic.

2 SERVINGS

INGREDIENTS

¾ cup shredded chicken from roasted chicken

3 tablespoons Buffalo Ranch Sauce (recipe in this book)

1 whole-wheat pizza ball

2 tablespoons fresh mozzarella

METHOD

1. Place your pizza stone in the oven and preheat it to the highest temperature possible. The pizza stone should be in the oven for at least an hour before putting the pizza in.

2. Stretch out the pizza dough into a 12-inch round. Instructions for dough preparation can be found in this book. Be sure to flour both sides of the dough generously to prevent sticking.

3. Once the dough is formed, move it onto the pizza peel. Quickly and evenly spread 1 tablespoon of Buffalo Ranch Sauce over the top of the dough, leaving the crust uncovered. Slide the pizza onto the preheated pizza stone.

4. Cook on the pizza stone for a few minutes (the time will vary depending on the heat of your oven) until the sauce begins to dry out slightly and the crust puffs up.

5. Add 2 tablespoons of Buffalo Ranch Sauce to the shredded chicken and stir to combine well.

6. Remove the pizza from the oven using the pizza peel. Scatter the shredded chicken evenly around the pizza. Scatter the mozzarella evenly over the pizza.

7. Return the pizza to the oven and cook until the cheese is crispy.

8. Remove the pizza from the oven, slice, and enjoy!

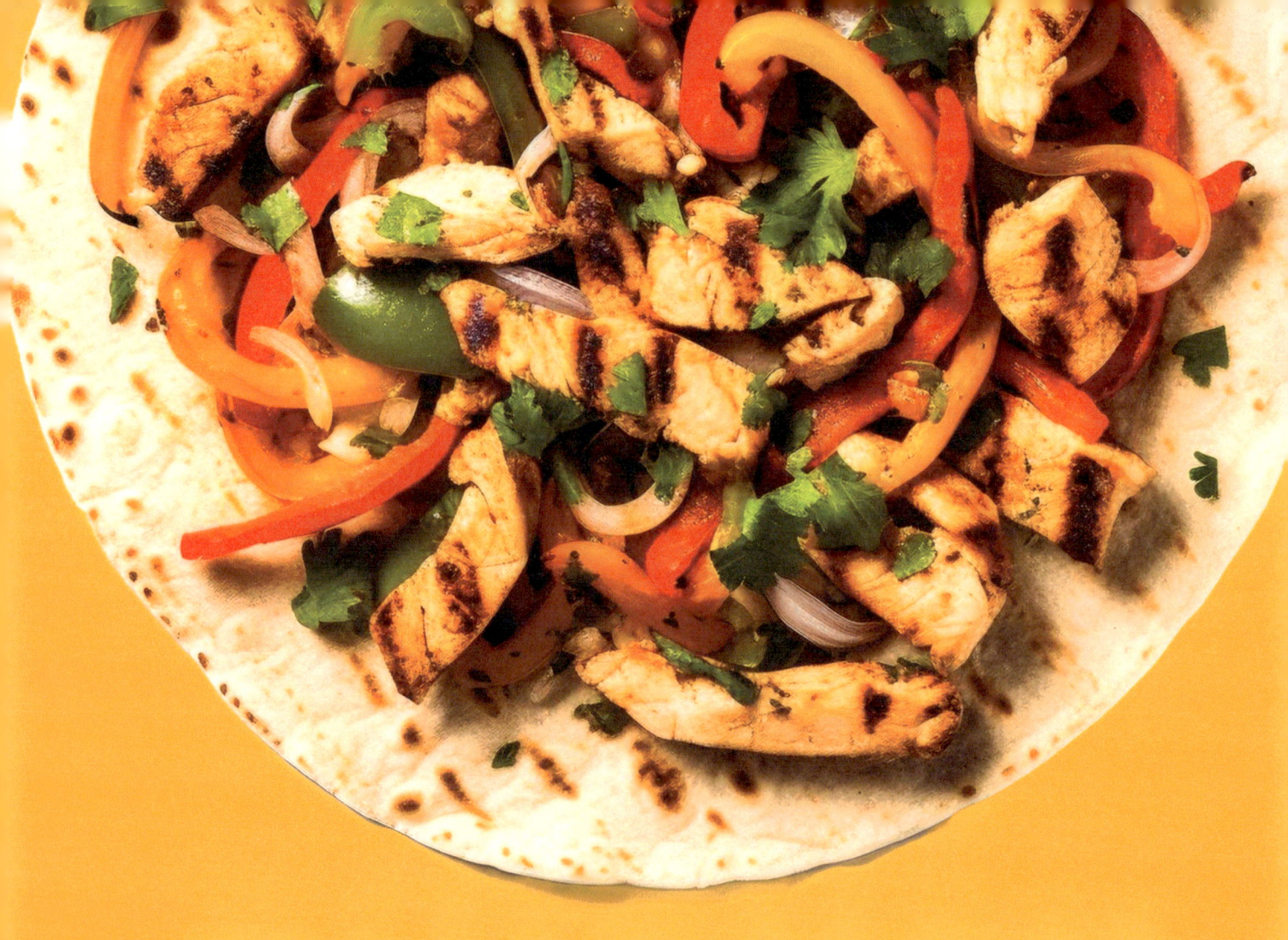

CHICKEN FAJITA

CHICKEN FAJITAS

These sizzling chicken fajitas are loaded with flavor. Perfect for a fun, tasty dinner.

INGREDIENTS

1 pound chicken breasts, sliced into strips

2 tablespoons chili powder

1 tablespoon garlic powder

1 tablespoon onion powder

1 tablespoon cumin

1 tablespoon ground coriander

1 chicken bouillon cube, crushed

2 tablespoons olive oil

1 green bell pepper, sliced into ribbons (seeds and white pith removed)

1 large yellow onion, sliced thin

2 cloves garlic, sliced thin

5 whole-wheat tortillas

1 tablespoon avocado oil

1 teaspoon soy sauce

1 recipe of guacamole (optional, recipe in this book)

Salt to taste

Total Servings	5
Per Serving	
Calories	383.6
Added Sugar	0g
Fiber	9.5g
Fat	14.5g
Saturated Fat	2.6g
Protein	33.8g

Values are approximate and does not include optional guacamole

METHOD

1. In a small bowl, combine chili powder, garlic powder, onion powder, cumin, ground coriander, and crushed chicken bouillon. Add olive oil to the bowl and stir to form a paste. Reserve 1 tablespoon of the paste for later. Add the chicken to the remaining paste and mix until thoroughly combined. Let marinate for as long as desired.

2. Heat a cast iron pan until it is very hot. Once hot, add the avocado oil, then add the marinated chicken to the pan. Cook the chicken on one side until it develops a nice color, then flip each piece and cook for about 30 seconds more. Transfer the chicken to a bowl.

3. Add a bit more avocado oil to the pan and add the onions. Add salt and cook until translucent. While the onions are cooking, heat up the tortillas in the microwave for 20 seconds. Optionally, spread some guacamole on each tortilla.

4. Once the onions are translucent, add the green peppers and cook until they start to brown. Add the sliced garlic and cook for 30 seconds. Add the reserved tablespoon of seasoning paste and cook for another 30 seconds.

5. Add the chicken back to the pan, stir, and add soy sauce.

6. Add some of the fajita mixture to each tortilla and enjoy!

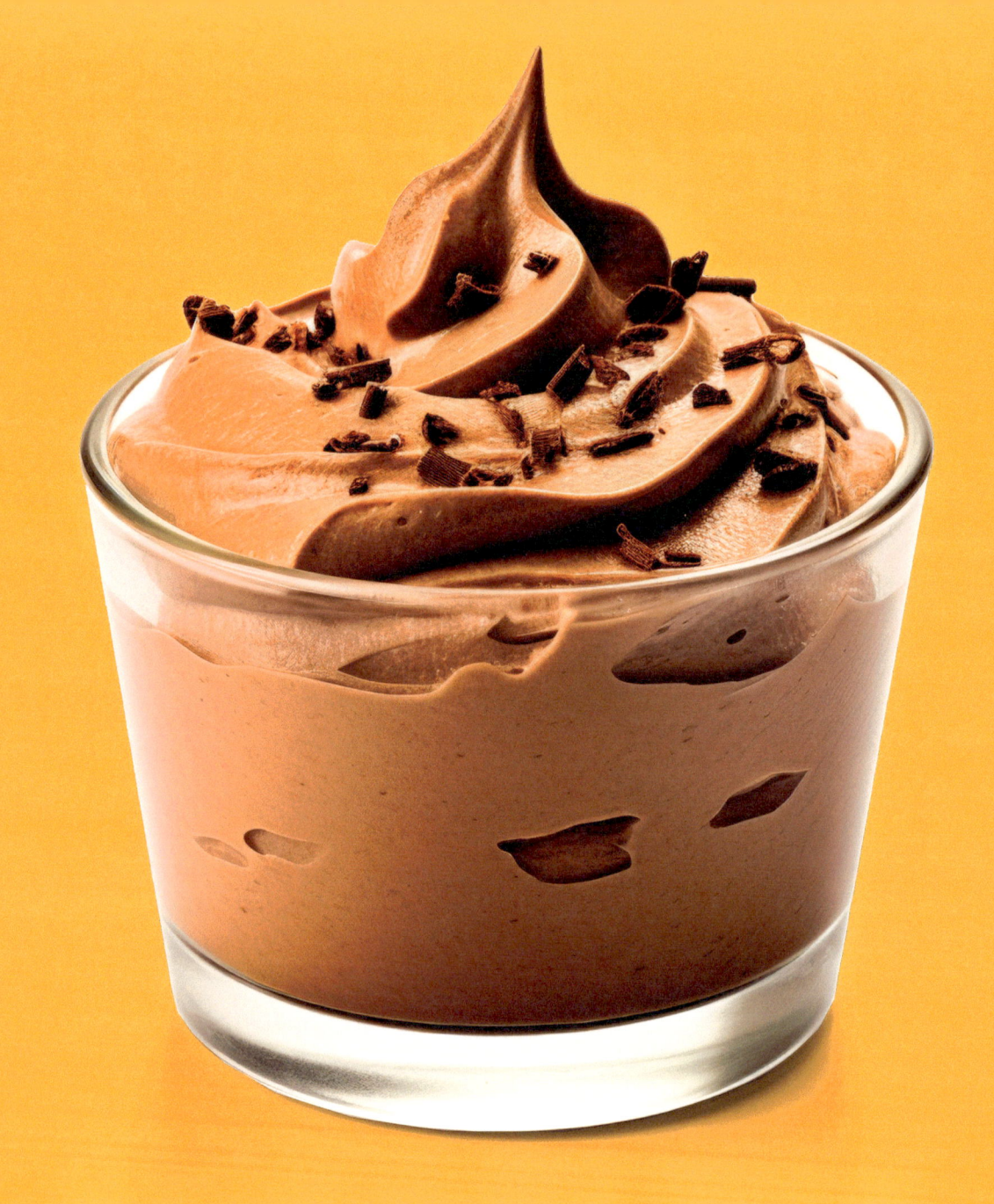

CHOCOLATE MOUSSE

CHOCOLATE MOUSSE

Rich, creamy chocolate mousse that's perfect for any chocoholic. Treat yourself!

INGREDIENTS

1 cup coconut non-fat milk

½ cup coconut oil

⅔ cup pure maple syrup

1 cup unsweetened cocoa powder

1 teaspoon vanilla extract

Pinch of sea salt

METHOD

1. Line an 8x8 inch baking pan with parchment paper, leaving some overhang on the sides for easy removal.

2. In a medium saucepan, combine the coconut non-fat milk, coconut oil, and maple syrup. Heat over medium heat until everything is melted and well combined.

3. Once the mixture is smooth, whisk in the cocoa powder until no lumps remain.

4. Stir in the vanilla extract and a pinch of sea salt. Mix until everything is well incorporated.

5. Pour the mixture into the prepared baking pan, spreading it out evenly.

6. Place the pan in the refrigerator and let the mousse set for at least 2-3 hours, or until firm.

7. Enjoy!

Total Servings	9
Per Serving	
Calories	254.2
Added Sugar	16.1g
Fiber	2.4g
Fat	19.8g
Saturated Fat	16.8g
Protein	2.5g

Values are approximate and may vary based on ingredients used

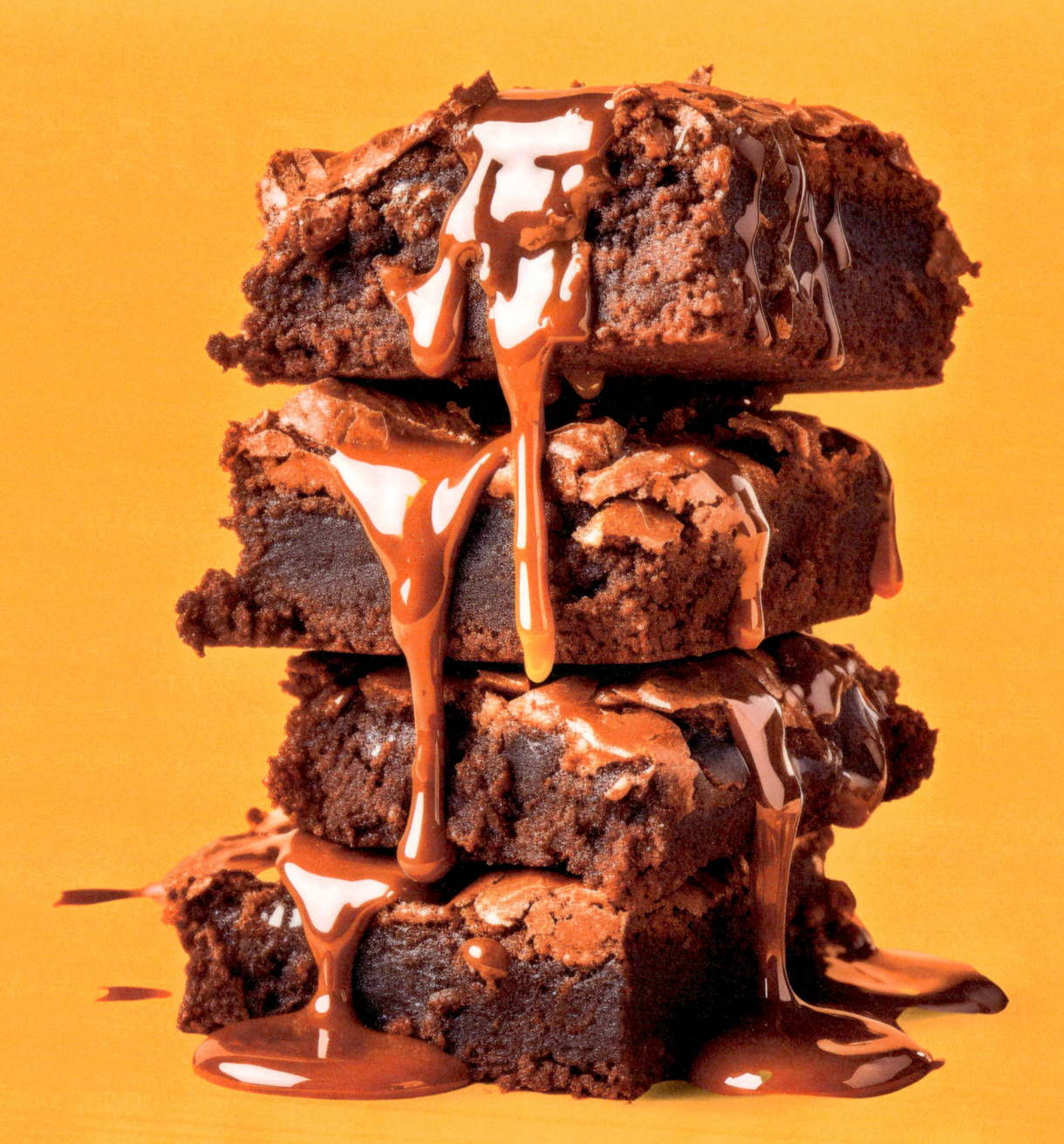

FLOURLESS BROWNIE

FLOURLESS BROWNIE

These fudgy, flourless brownies are gluten-free and totally delicious. A must-try for brownie lovers.

INGREDIENTS

6 tablespoons coconut oil

1 cup 70% cocoa chocolate chips

2 eggs

1 teaspoon vanilla extract

1 cup allulose

2 tablespoons cocoa powder

3 tablespoons arrowroot powder

METHOD

1. Preheat oven to 350°F and line an 8x8 inch baking tray with parchment paper.

2. Combine coconut oil and chocolate chips in a microwave-safe bowl. Microwave in 30-second intervals, stirring until the chocolate is melted. Let the mixture rest at room temperature for 5 minutes.

3. Whisk in the allulose until the batter is smooth and let it sit for a minute.

4. Whisk in the eggs, one at a time, until the texture is very smooth. Then whisk in the vanilla extract, cocoa powder, and arrowroot powder until the mixture is smooth and free of clumps.

5. Pour the batter into the prepared baking tray and bake in the oven for 20 minutes for a fudgy texture, or up to 25 minutes for a firmer texture.

6. Enjoy!

Total Servings	12
Per Serving	
Calories	146.6
Added Sugar	3.4g
Fiber	1.3g
Fat	12.4g
Saturated Fat	9.3g
Protein	1.9g

Values are approximate and may vary based on ingredients used

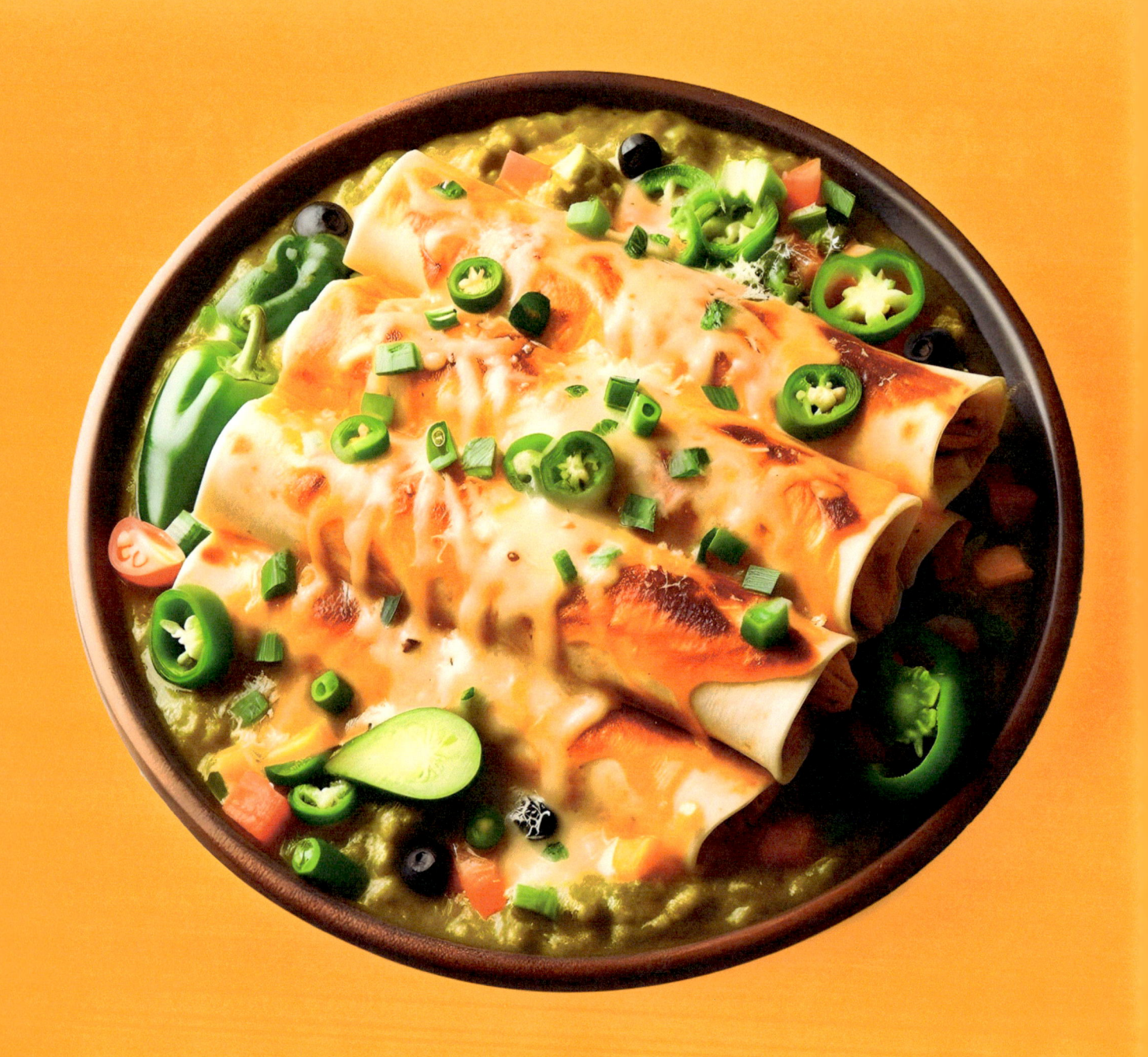

GREEN CHILLI ENCHILADAS

GREEN CHILE ENCHILADAS

Spice up dinner with these green chile enchiladas. They're packed with flavor and super satisfying.

INGREDIENTS

2 cups shredded chicken

½ white onion, diced

5 whole-wheat tortillas

7 poblano chiles

7 tomatillos

½ cup non-fat milk

2 cups chicken broth

1 cup low-fat mozzarella

Salt and pepper to taste

Total Servings	5
Per Serving	
Calories	299.2
Added Sugar	0g
Fiber	8.8g
Fat	6.9g
Saturated Fat	2.4g
Protein	27.3g

Values are approximate and may vary based on ingredients used

Note: *Use tongs and gloves when roasting chiles or handling hot cookware to avoid burns.*

METHOD

1. Preheat oven to 380°F.
2. If you have a gas stove, place each poblano chile directly on a high flame. Turn the chile with tongs until the entire surface is blackened. Once blackened, place the chile in a bowl and cover with a lid. Repeat for all chiles. Alternatively, roast the chiles in the oven at 450°F until the skin is blackened. Then place them in a bowl and cover with a lid to steam for a few minutes. After steaming, rub off the skin under cold water and deseed the chiles. Set aside.
3. Boil the tomatillos in water for about 10 minutes. Once done, add them to a blender along with the roasted poblanos and chicken broth. Blend until smooth.
4. Pour the blended sauce into a saucepan and season with salt and pepper to taste. Heat gently over medium heat.
5. Ladle some of the sauce into the bottom of a medium-small casserole dish.
6. Microwave the tortillas for 10 seconds to soften them.
7. Dip each tortilla in the sauce from the saucepan, then add some shredded chicken, diced onion, and mozzarella inside the tortilla. Wrap it up and place it in the casserole dish. Repeat for all tortillas, laying them side by side in the dish.
8. Pour the remaining sauce over the enchiladas in the casserole dish.
9. Sprinkle the remaining mozzarella over the top of the enchiladas.
10. Bake in the oven for about 20 minutes or until the cheese is melted on top.
11. Enjoy!

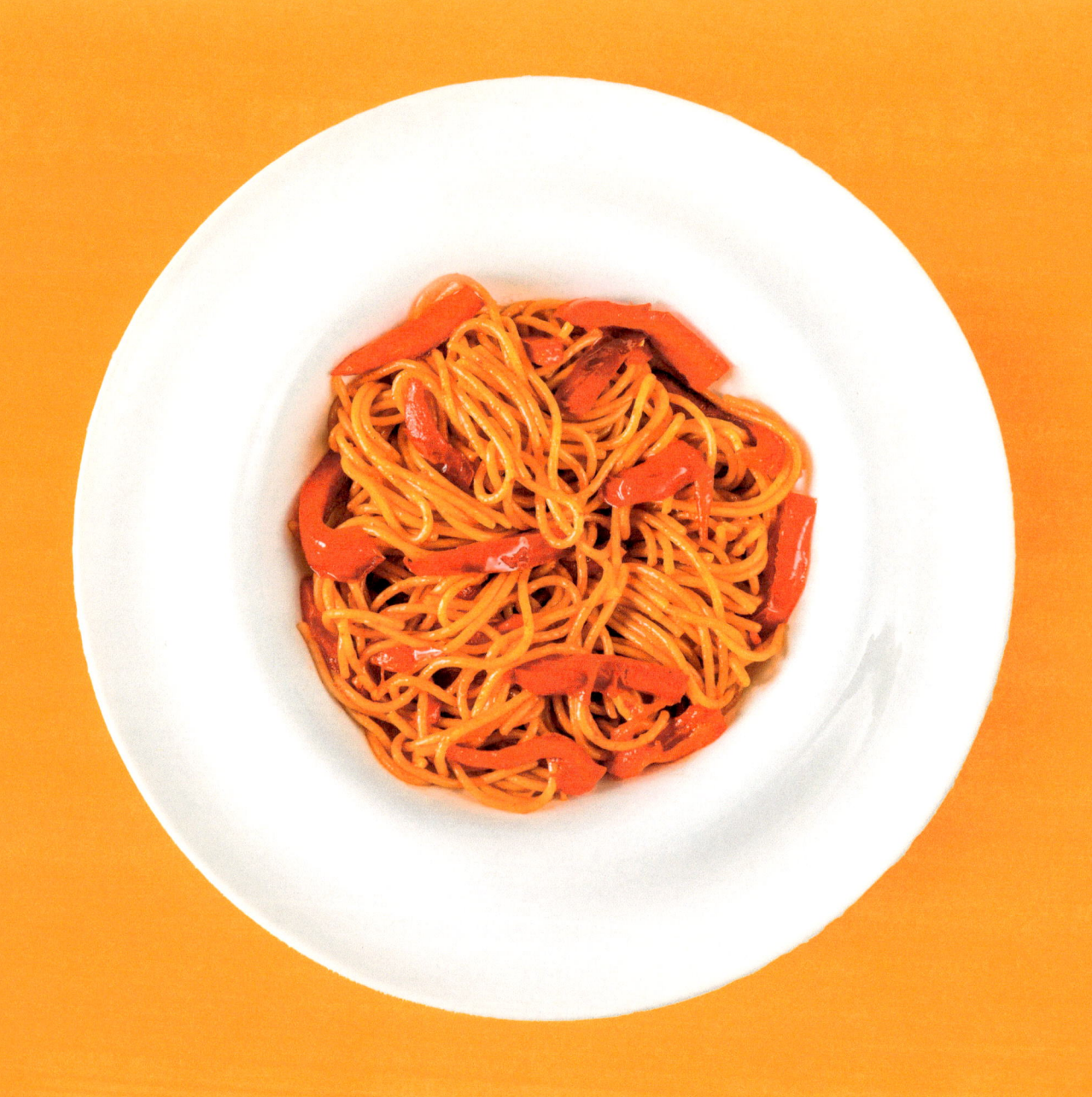

ROASTED PEPPER PASTA

ROASTED PEPPER PASTA

This roasted pepper pasta is seriously delicious and packed with flavor. You'll love it!

INGREDIENTS

1 red pepper

2 calabrian chiles, seeded with ½ tablespoon of liquid they are stored in (use 3 if you want it really spicy)

½ teaspoon red pepper flakes

2 garlic cloves, sliced thin

1 tablespoon tomato paste

8 oz chickpea cavatappi pasta

½ yellow onion, sliced thin

1 tablespoon olive oil

½ cup cauliflower

1 cup non-fat milk

Salt to taste

Pecorino Romano to taste

Total Servings	2
Per Serving	
Calories	579.4
Added Sugar	0g
Fiber	14g
Fat	11.1g
Saturated Fat	1.5g
Protein	27.6g
Values are approximate and may vary based on ingredients used	

Note: *Use tongs and handle hot things with caution.*

METHOD

1. Add cauliflower and non-fat milk to a pot and bring to a boil. Cook the cauliflower until it is mushy. Once mushy, add it to a blender with enough of the non-fat milk from the pot to form the consistency of heavy cream. Blend and set aside.

2. Place the red pepper directly over a gas flame or under a broiler, turning until the skin is blackened all over. Place the roasted pepper in a bowl and cover with a lid to steam for a few minutes. After steaming, rub off the skin under cold water, then deseed and devein the pepper. Cut it into strips and set aside.

3. In a medium saucepan, add olive oil and heat over medium. Add the onions with a little salt and stir occasionally until they start to caramelize.

4. Start boiling water for the pasta.

5. Once the onions start to caramelize, add the roasted pepper strips and cook until they begin to soften. Add the garlic, calabrian chilis, tomato paste, and red pepper flakes and cook for about a minute.

6. Add the chickpea cavatappi pasta to the boiling water and cook according to package instructions.

7. To the pan with the peppers and onions, add about ½ cup of the cauliflower blended mixture and a little bit of pasta water. Stir and cook for 30 seconds, then transfer this mixture to a blender and blend until very smooth.

8. Pour half of the blended sauce back into the pan. Reserve ½ cup of pasta water, then strain the pasta.

9. Add half of the reserved pasta water to the pan, then add half of the cooked pasta noodles and stir to combine. Cook for 30 seconds.

10. Plate the pasta and top with Pecorino Romano. This dish serves two, so repeat the pasta water and sauce method for the second portion.

11. Enjoy!

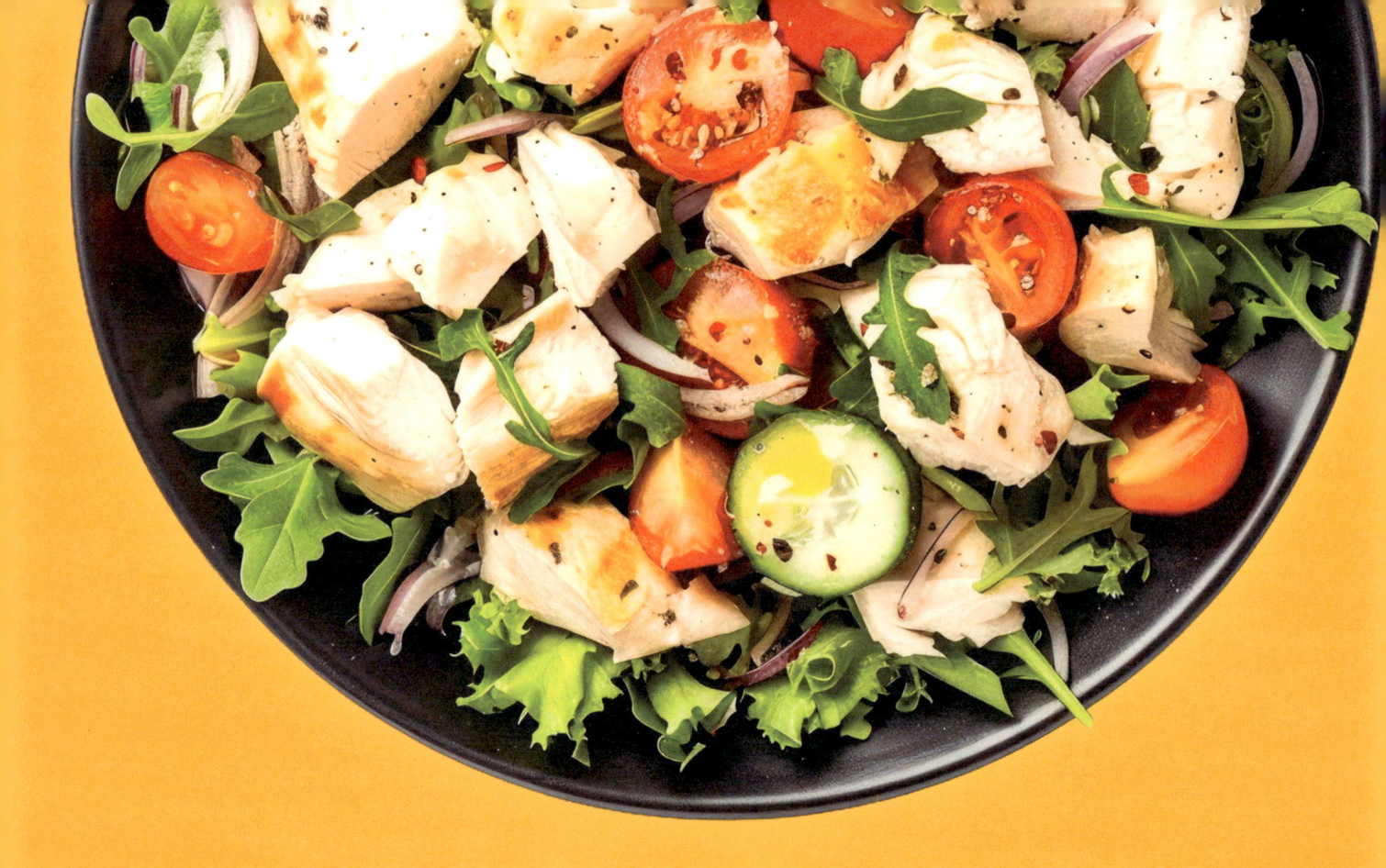

THE BEST CHICKEN SALAD EVER

THE BEST CHICKEN SALAD EVER

This chicken salad is amazing. Flavorful, fresh, and perfect for sandwiches or on its own.

INGREDIENTS

2 chicken breasts, chopped into cubes

1 teaspoon salt

½ teaspoon garlic powder

½ teaspoon smoked paprika

½ teaspoon black pepper

1 teaspoon avocado oil

2 pickle wedges, diced

1.5 tablespoons tomato, diced

1.5 tablespoons red onion, diced

3 tablespoons light mayonnaise

1.5 tablespoons stone ground mustard

4 dashes Tabasco sauce

METHOD

1. Season the chicken breasts with salt, garlic powder, smoked paprika, and black pepper.

2. Heat avocado oil in a pan over medium-high heat. Once the pan is really hot, add the seasoned chicken. Cook for 3 minutes without flipping, then flip and cook until the chicken is cooked through. Remove from heat and set aside for 5 minutes.

3. Chop the chicken into smaller pieces.

4. In a bowl, combine the chopped chicken, pickles, tomato, red onion, light mayonnaise, mustard, and Tabasco sauce. Mix well.

5. Refrigerate the mixture for 30 minutes.

6. Take it out and enjoy!

Total Servings	2
Per Serving	
Calories	303
Added Sugar	0g
Fiber	1.3g
Fat	11.5g
Saturated Fat	2.0g
Protein	41.0g

Values are approximate and may vary based on ingredients used

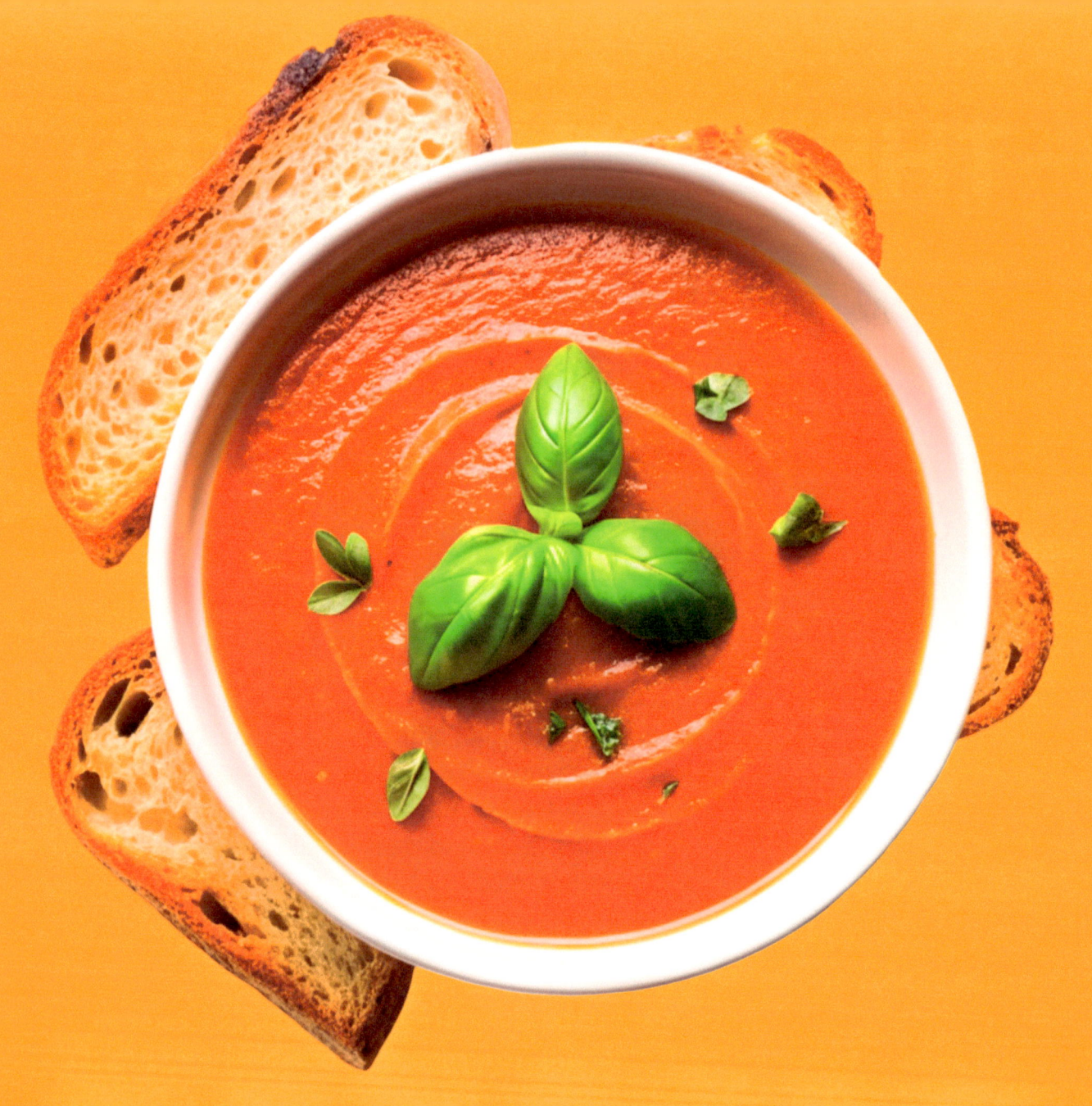

ROASTED TOMATO SOUP

ROASTED TOMATO SOUP

Warm up with this rich, comforting roasted tomato soup. Perfect for a cozy meal at home.

INGREDIENTS

11 Roma tomatoes, cut in half

10 garlic cloves, with skins on

1 bulb fennel, core removed and cut up

5 tablespoons paprika

2 cups V8 juice

2 cups vegetable stock

1 bunch thyme

2 bay leaves

1 bunch of basil

1 onion, diced

2 carrots, diced

2 celery stalks, diced

2 tablespoons olive oil

Salt to taste

Pepper to taste

METHOD

1. Preheat oven to 450°F.
2. Place Roma tomatoes, garlic cloves, and fennel on a baking tray. Drizzle with 1 tablespoon of olive oil, season with salt and pepper, and toss to coat. Roast in the oven for 20-25 minutes.
3. While the vegetables are roasting, heat the remaining tablespoon of olive oil in a large pot over medium heat. Add the diced carrots, celery, and onion with a pinch of salt. Cook, stirring occasionally, for 10 minutes.
4. Once the vegetables are done roasting, add the tomatoes and fennel to the pot. Squeeze the roasted garlic out of its skins and add to the pot.
5. Add the paprika, thyme, and bay leaves to the pot, stirring to combine. Cook for 5 minutes.
6. Pour in the V8 juice and vegetable stock. Bring to a simmer and cook for 30 minutes.
7. Remove the bay leaves and thyme stems. Transfer the soup to a blender and blend until smooth.
8. Return the blended soup to the pot. Add the basil leaves and stir to combine. If the soup is too thick, add more vegetable stock to reach the desired consistency.
9. Simmer the soup for at least an hour, stirring occasionally. The longer it cooks, the better the flavors will develop.
10. Before serving, remove the basil leaves.
11. Enjoy!

Total Servings	6
Per Serving	
Calories	159
Added Sugar	0g
Fiber	9.8g
Fat	6.2g
Saturated Fat	1.0g
Protein	5.4g

Values are approximate and may vary based on ingredients used

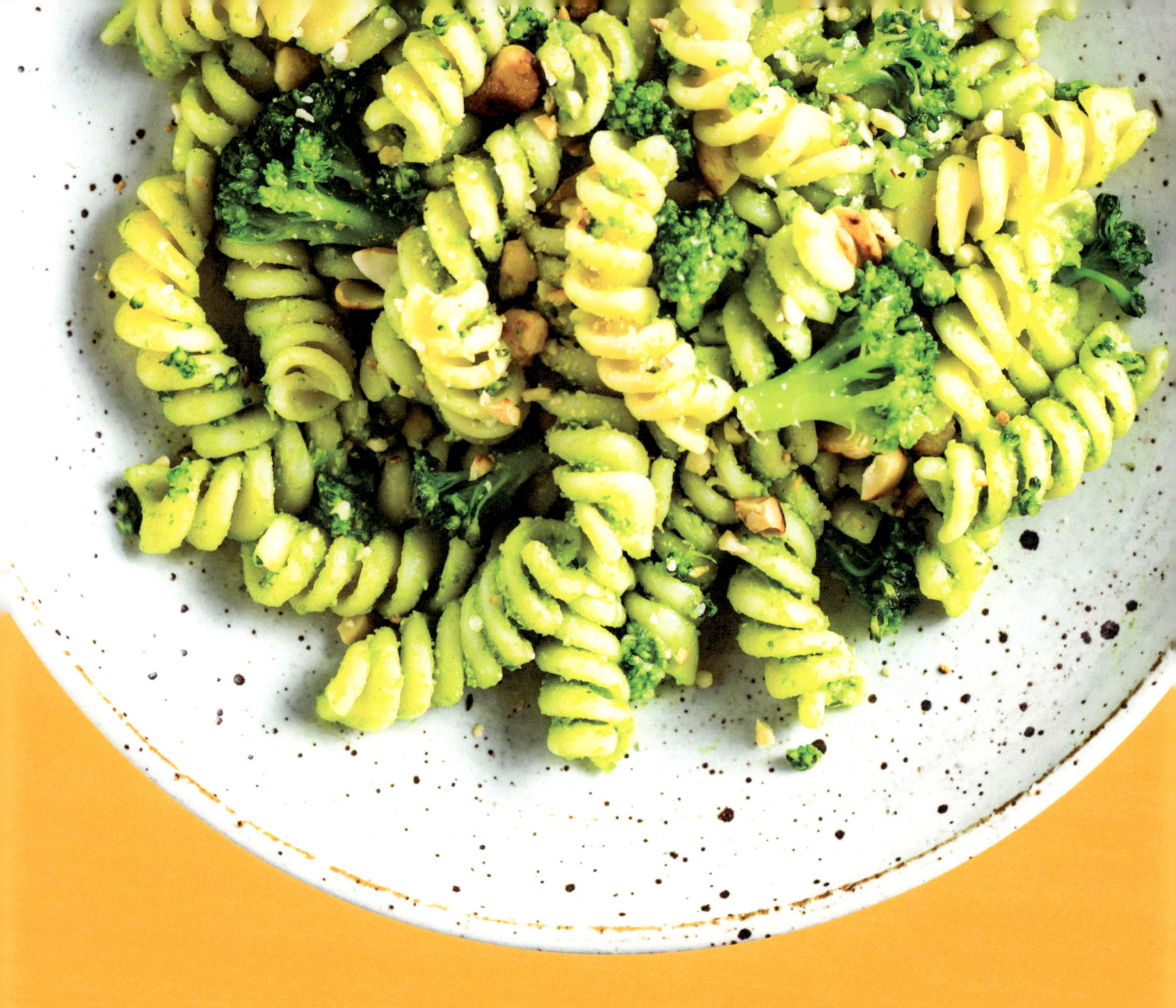

CREAMY
BROCCOLI PASTA

CREAMY BROCCOLI PASTA

Get your veggies in with this creamy broccoli pasta. It's healthy, delicious, and super satisfying.

INGREDIENTS

3 large broccoli heads with stems (shave the stems until they are no longer rough)

3 cloves garlic, sliced thin

2 teaspoons chili flakes

2 tablespoons olive oil (1 for roasting and 1 for cooking)

1 pound healthy pasta (e.g., chickpea penne pasta)

¼ cup Pecorino Romano

METHOD

1. Preheat oven to 500°F. Set a pot of water to boil.

2. Cut the florets of 2 broccoli heads into even, smaller florets and lay them out on a baking sheet. Coat with 1 tablespoon of olive oil and roast for 10 minutes.

3. Meanwhile, cut up the stems and remaining florets of those 2 broccoli heads, as well as the entire third broccoli head, into thin pieces. Add them all to the boiling water and boil for 10 minutes. Preserve some of the boiling water.

4. In a saucepan, heat 1 tablespoon of olive oil over medium heat. Once hot, add the garlic and chili flakes and cook until lightly browned. Add the boiled broccoli and mash it with a wooden spoon. Add some of the preserved water to the saucepan to help mash the broccoli.

5. Start another pot of water to boil for the pasta. Once boiling, add salt and the pasta, cooking for a minute less than the lowest recommended time for al dente.

6. While the pasta is cooking, blend the broccoli mixture from the saucepan until very smooth.

7. Add the blended broccoli sauce back to a pot. Stir in ½ cup of pasta water to the sauce and combine. Adjust seasoning to taste.

8. Add the cooked pasta to the sauce and stir, cooking for 30 seconds. Stir in the Pecorino Romano and cook for an additional 30 seconds.

9. Plate the pasta and top with some of the roasted broccoli florets.

10. Enjoy!

Total Servings	4
Per Serving	
Calories	308.5
Added Sugar	0g
Fiber	9.1g
Fat	11.5g
Saturated Fat	2.6g
Protein	18.1g

Values are approximate and may vary based on ingredients used

DOUBLE
CHESSEBURGER

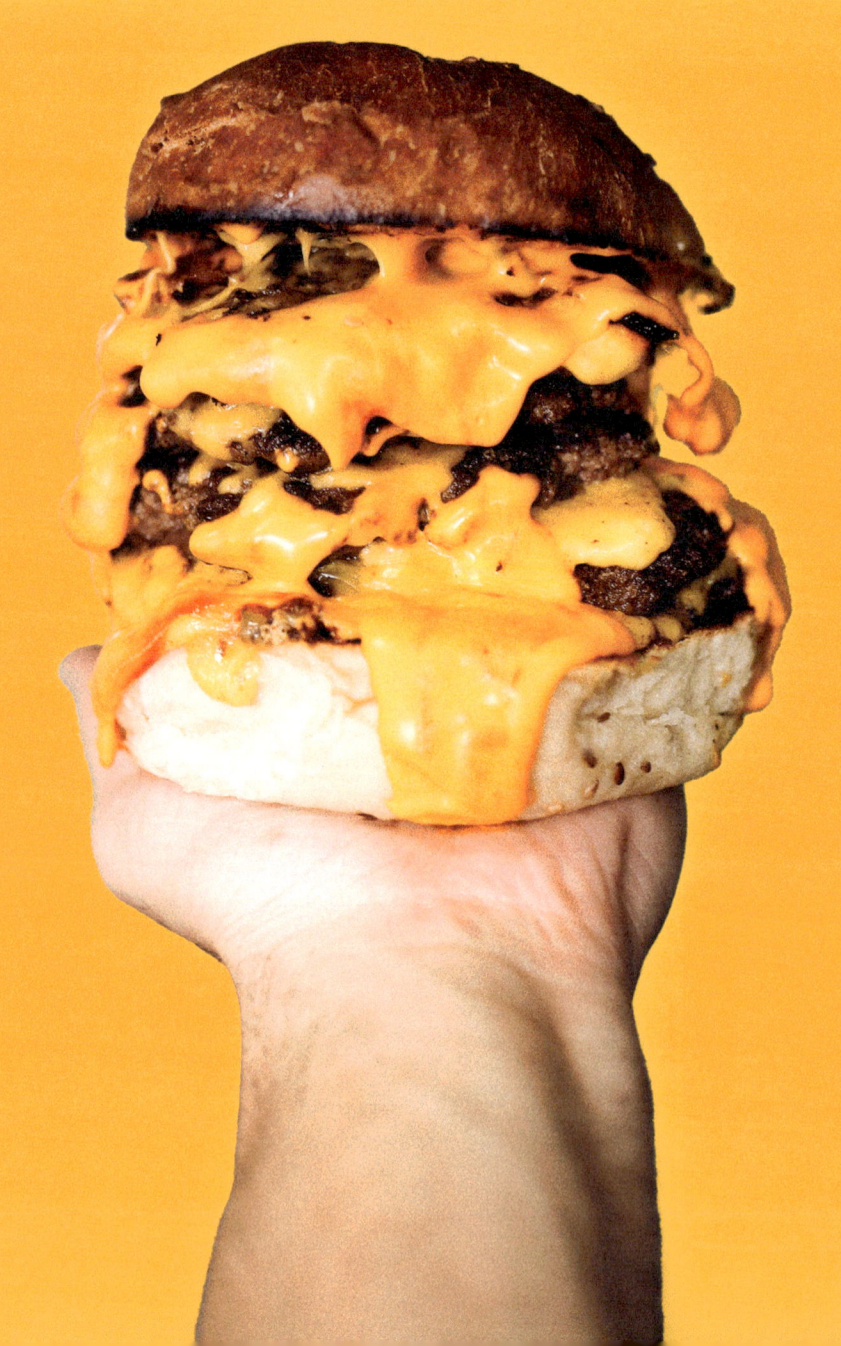

DOUBLE CHEESEBURGER

Indulge in this epic double cheeseburger. Loaded with flavor and perfect for satisfying your burger cravings.

INGREDIENTS

2 3oz balls of the leanest beef you can find

2 slices of low-fat or non-fat American cheese

1 tablespoon low-fat mayo

1 tablespoon ketchup

½ tablespoon sriracha

1 whole-wheat burger bun

1 teaspoon canola oil

2 pinches of salt

2 pinches of black pepper

Pinch of turmeric

METHOD

1. Combine mayo, ketchup, and sriracha in a small bowl.

2. Toast the burger bun in a toaster oven.

3. Heat up a cast iron pan and add canola oil. Once very hot, smash one beef patty very thin and season with a pinch of salt, a pinch of pepper, and a pinch of turmeric. Cook for 2 minutes or until the bottom is crispy, then flip and cook for 10 seconds. Add a slice of American cheese, cover with a lid, and let the cheese melt for 1 minute. Remove the patty from the pan.

4. Repeat the same process for the second patty.

5. Spread a tablespoon of the sauce on the bottom of the toasted bun, add the patties, and top with the other half of the bun.

6. Enjoy!

Total Servings	1
Per Serving	
Calories	616.5
Added Sugar	4.2g
Fiber	3.3g
Fat	29g
Saturated Fat	9.9g
Protein	56.4g

Values are approximate and may vary based on ingredients used

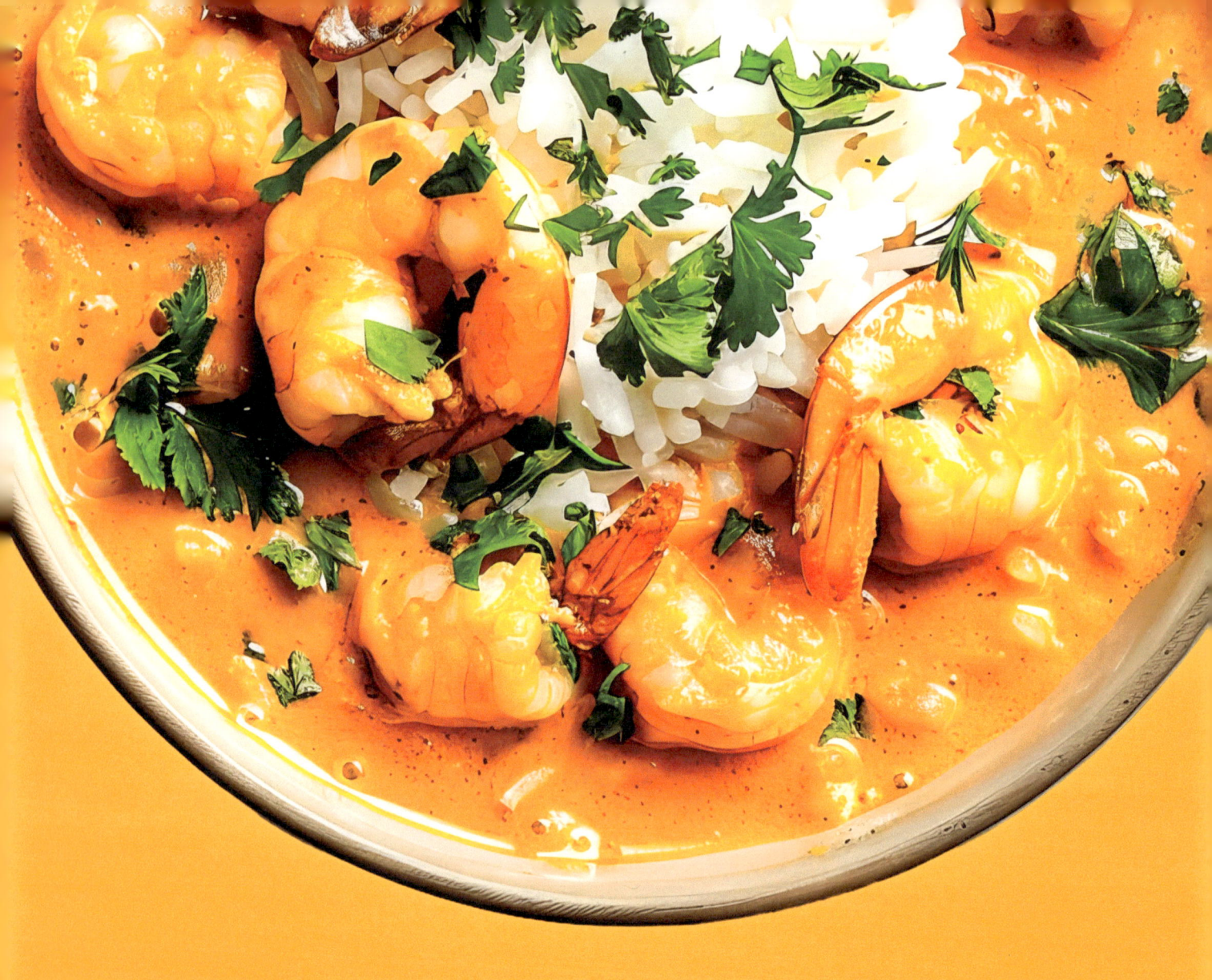

SHRIMP CURRY

SHRIMP CURRY

Take your taste buds on a trip with this flavorful shrimp curry. Spicy, creamy, and absolutely delicious.

INGREDIENTS

½ pound shrimp

Pinch of salt

Pinch of pepper

Pinch of cayenne pepper

1 teaspoon lemon juice

½ tablespoon canola oil

½ medium yellow onion, diced

2 cloves garlic, minced

½ tablespoon grated ginger

¼ teaspoon black pepper

½ teaspoon turmeric

1 teaspoon ground coriander

½ teaspoon curry powder

7.5 oz diced tomatoes with juice

7 oz coconut non-fat milk

METHOD

1. Combine shrimp, salt, pepper, cayenne pepper, and lemon juice in a bowl. Let marinate for 10 minutes.

2. While the shrimp is marinating, heat the oil in a medium-sized skillet. Add the diced onion and cook for 2-3 minutes until the onion softens and becomes translucent.

3. Stir in the garlic, ginger, black pepper, salt, coriander, turmeric, and curry powder. Cook for another minute.

4. Add the diced tomatoes with their juices and the coconut non-fat milk. Stir and bring to a boil. Cook for about 5 minutes, stirring occasionally.

5. Add the shrimp along with the accumulated juices from the marinade. Cook for another 2 minutes, or until the shrimp is pink and cooked through.

6. Enjoy!

Total Servings	2
Per Serving	
Calories	261.4
Added Sugar	0g
Fiber	2.7g
Fat	12.6g
Saturated Fat	6.7g
Protein	25.1g

Values are approximate and may vary based on ingredients used

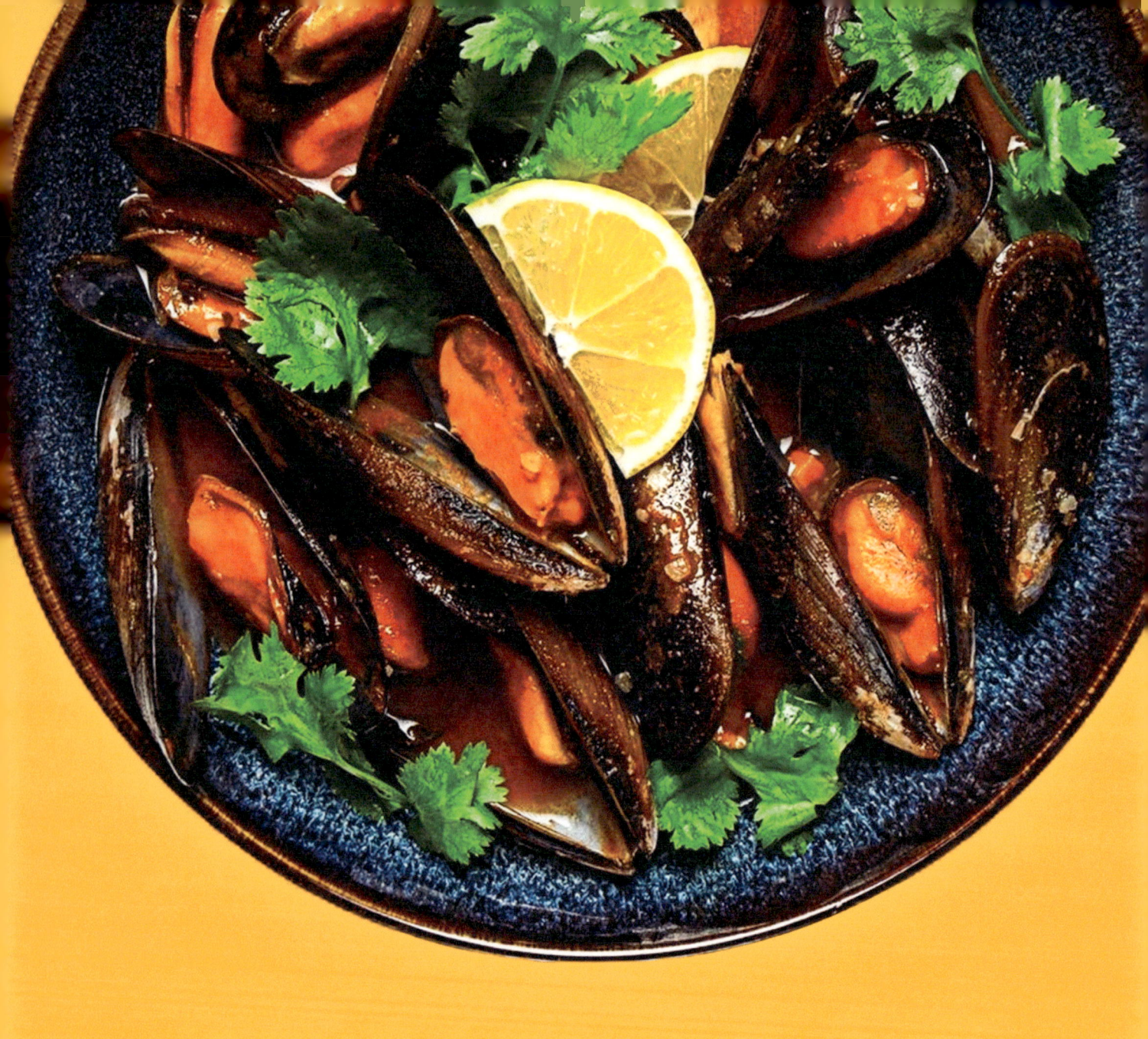

MUSSELS FRA DIAVOLO

MUSSELS FRA DIAVOLO

Spicy, flavorful mussels fra diavolo is a seafood dish that's sure to impress. Perfect for a special dinner.

INGREDIENTS

1 bag of mussels, cleaned and debearded

1 24 oz can of whole peeled tomatoes, blended

½ yellow onion, minced very fine

2 large cloves of garlic, sliced thin

10 basil leaves

1 teaspoon dried oregano

2 teaspoons chili flakes

2-3 Calabrian chilis, deseeded (depending on spice preference)

1 cup white wine

Juice from ½ lemon

2 tablespoons olive oil

METHOD

1. Add olive oil to a large saucepan and heat over medium. Add the onions and cook for a couple of minutes or until they soften. Once softened, add garlic, chili flakes, basil leaves, and oregano. Cook for 1 minute, then add the Calabrian chilis. Cook for another 30 seconds.

2. Add the white wine to deglaze the pan. Once the wine has reduced, add the blended tomatoes.

3. Reduce the tomatoes over medium heat until they are very thick.

4. Once the sauce is thick, add the mussels and stir to combine. Cover with a lid and cook for 1 minute and 30 seconds. Open the lid and check if the mussels are half open. If they are, turn off the heat, add the rest of the basil leaves, stir, and cover the lid for another 30 seconds.

5. Squeeze lemon juice on top, plate, and enjoy!

Total Servings	3
Per Serving	
Calories	318.7
Added Sugar	0g
Fiber	4.5g
Fat	11.9g
Saturated Fat	1.9g
Protein	19.2g

Values are approximate and may vary based on ingredients used

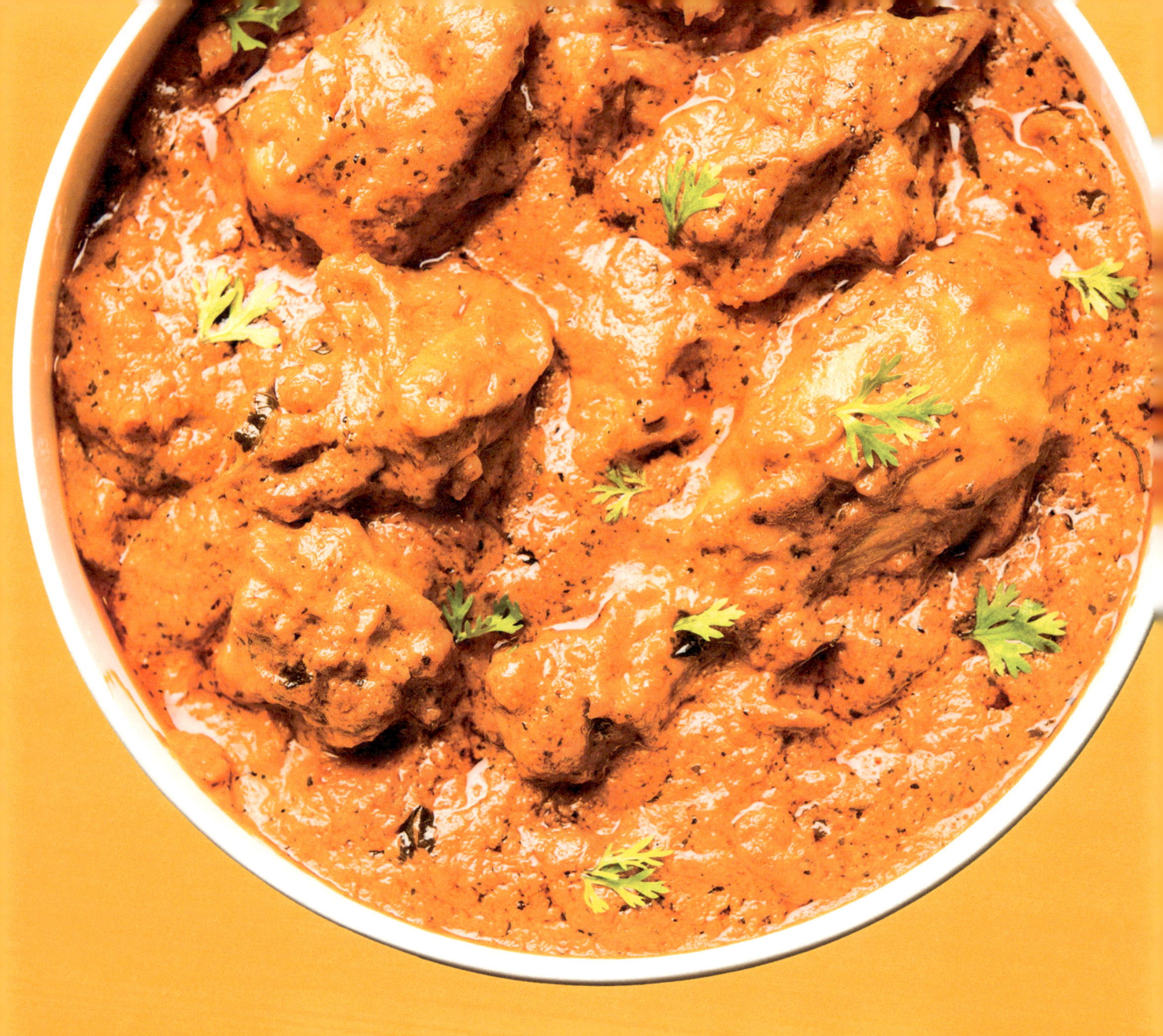

BUTTER CHICKEN

BUTTER CHICKEN

Indulge in this rich, creamy butter chicken. It's a classic Indian dish that's perfect for dinner.

INGREDIENTS

For marinade:

2 pounds chicken thighs, cubed

¾ cup yogurt

1.5 tablespoons garlic paste

1 tablespoon ginger paste

2 teaspoons salt

2 teaspoons garam masala

1 teaspoon turmeric

2 teaspoons chili powder

For sauce:

1 tablespoon ghee

1 medium yellow onion, diced

3 cloves garlic, minced

1 teaspoon grated ginger

1 tablespoon garam masala

2.5 teaspoons chili powder

1.5 teaspoons turmeric

1 tablespoon tomato paste

14 oz diced tomatoes (canned)

½ cup cashews

1 cup non-fat (skim) milk

METHOD

1. Combine chicken, yogurt, garlic paste, ginger paste, salt, garam masala, turmeric, and chili powder in a bowl. Marinate in the fridge for as long as you like (the longer, the better, up to 2 days).

2. Heat ½ tablespoon ghee in a large saucepan over medium heat. Add the marinated chicken and cook for 3-4 minutes. Remove the chicken and set aside.

3. Add another ½ tablespoon ghee to the same saucepan and heat over medium. Add the diced onion and cook for 4 minutes, constantly scraping the bottom of the pan, with add the diced onion, garam masala, chili powder, and turmeric, and cook for 4 minutes, constantly scraping the bottom of the pan.

4. Add the minced garlic and grated ginger and cook for another 3 minutes.

5. Stir in the tomato paste, diced tomatoes, cashews, and non-fat milk. Cook for 3 minutes, scraping the bottom of the pan.

6. Transfer everything in the saucepan to a blender and blend until smooth.

7. Return the blended sauce to the saucepan and add the cooked chicken. Simmer for about 15 minutes.

8. Enjoy!

Total Servings	4
Per Serving	
Calories	345.8
Added Sugar	0g
Fiber	3.2g
Fat	22.0g
Saturated Fat	6.1g
Protein	24.7g

Values are approximate and may vary based on ingredients used

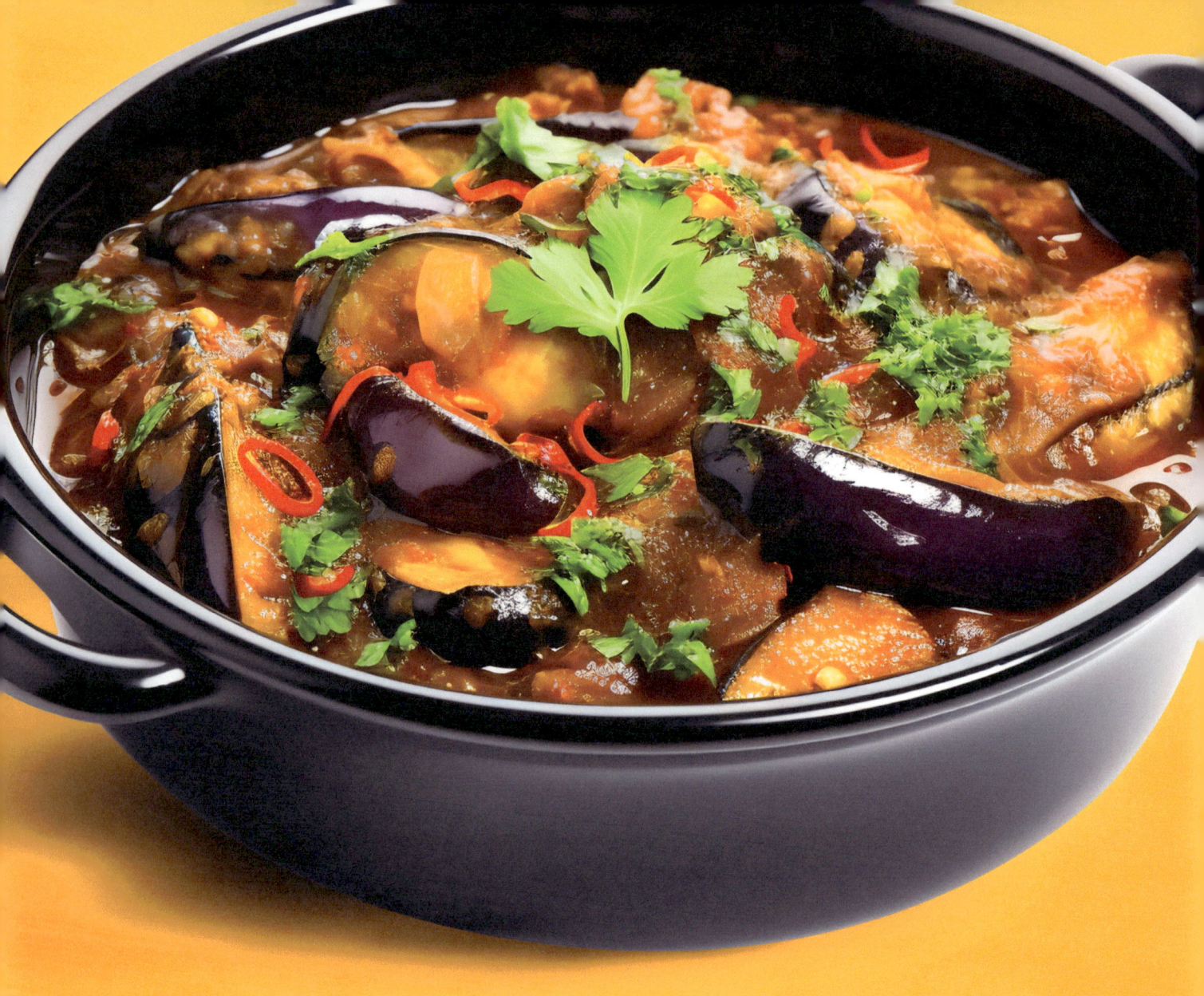

BAINGAN BARTHA

BAINGAN BARTHA

Experience the smoky, flavorful taste of baingan bartha. It's a delicious eggplant dish packed with flavor.

INGREDIENTS

1 lb eggplant

4 cloves garlic (for roasting), peeled

2 Thai green chilis, cut in half

1 tablespoon olive oil

½ cup yellow onion, diced

1 tomato, chopped and deseeded

3 garlic cloves (for sauce), chopped fine

1 teaspoon grated ginger

½ teaspoon garam masala

Total Servings	3
Per Serving	
Calories	117.8
Added Sugar	0g
Fiber	6.1g
Fat	5.0g
Saturated Fat	0.8g
Protein	3.1g

Values are approximate and may vary based on ingredients used

METHOD

1. Make 4 large slits in the eggplant. Insert 1 garlic clove and ½ a Thai green chili into each slit.

2. Roast the Eggplant: Place the eggplant directly over an open flame (gas stove or grill) and roast until the skin is charred and the flesh is soft, turning frequently for even roasting. This should take about 10-15 minutes. Alternatively, you can roast the eggplant in a 450°F oven for 20-25 minutes, turning occasionally.

3. Once roasted, place the eggplant in a bowl and cover it to steam. After 7 minutes, peel off the skin and remove the green top. Mash the eggplant in a bowl and set aside.

4. In a large saucepan, heat olive oil over medium heat. Add the yellow onion and a pinch of salt, cooking until the onion is soft.

5. Add the chopped garlic, grated ginger, chopped tomato, and garam masala to the saucepan. Add another pinch of salt and cook until the tomato is soft.

6. Add the mashed eggplant to the saucepan and cook for 3 minutes, stirring well to combine the flavors.

7. Plate and enjoy!

Note: *Use tongs and handle with caution.*

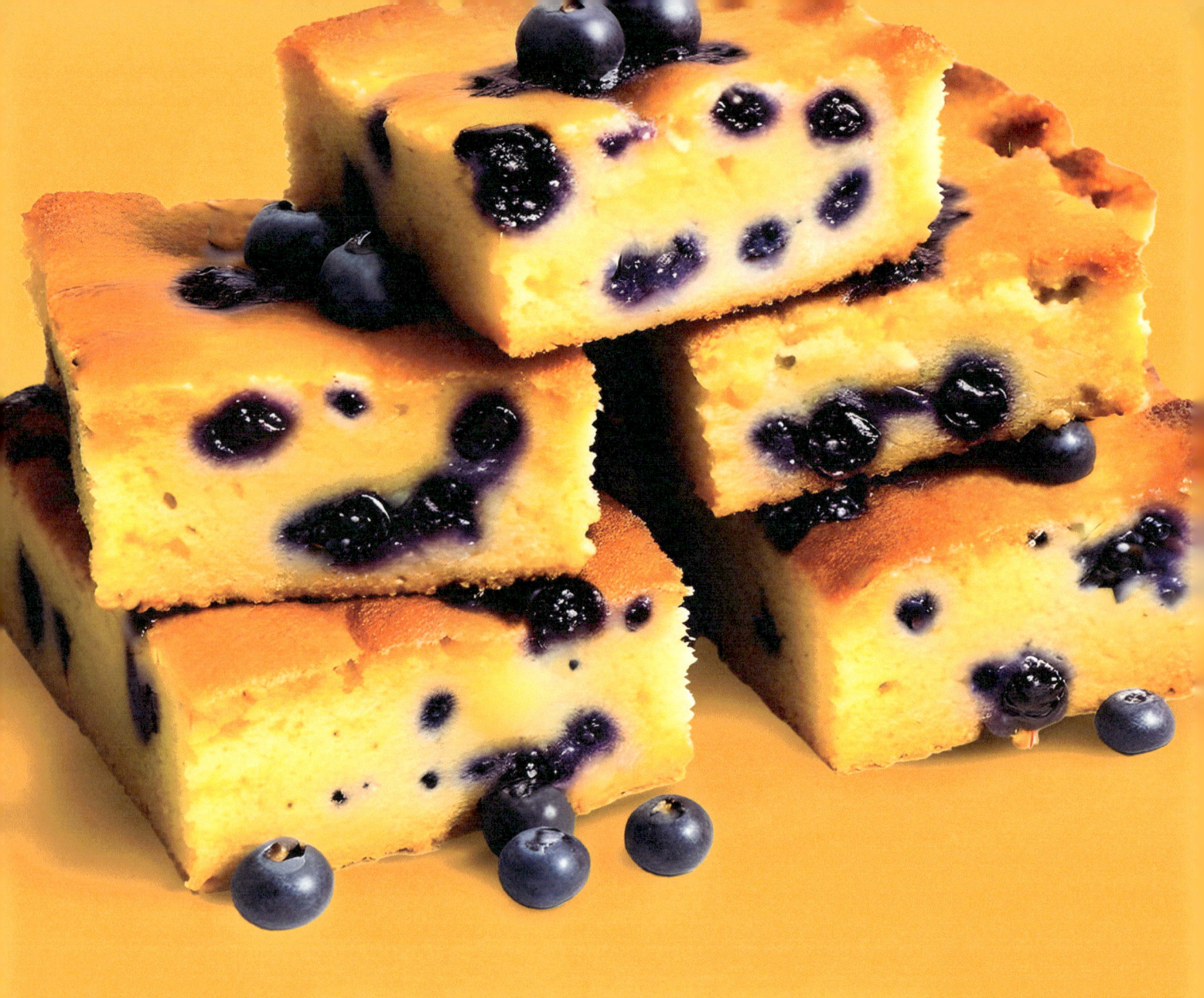

BLUEBERRY GLAZED CORNBREAD

BLUEBERRY GLAZED CORNBREAD

Treat yourself to this sweet, moist blueberry glazed cornbread. A delicious twist on a classic favorite.

INGREDIENTS

1.25 cups (150 g) cornmeal

½ cup (60 g) whole-wheat flour

1.5 teaspoons baking powder

½ teaspoon baking soda

¼ teaspoon salt

1 tablespoon coconut oil, melted and cooled

1 large egg, room temperature

1 teaspoon vanilla extract

½ cup non-fat Greek yogurt

¼ cup maple syrup

¼ cup non-fat milk

5 blueberries, mashed

1 tablespoon honey

2 tablespoons water

METHOD

1. Spray an 8 x 8 inch baking sheet with cooking spray and preheat the oven to 350°F.

2. In a medium bowl, whisk together the cornmeal, flour, baking powder, baking soda, and salt.

3. In a separate bowl, whisk together the coconut oil, egg, and vanilla. Stir in the Greek yogurt, mixing until no large lumps remain. Stir in the maple syrup.

4. Alternate between adding the cornmeal mixture and non-fat milk to the wet ingredients, beginning and ending with the cornmeal mixture, stirring just until incorporated. It is best to add the cornmeal mixture in 4 parts.

5. Spread the batter into the prepared pan. Bake at 350°F for 18-20 minutes or until the edges begin to turn golden and the center feels firm to the touch. Cool in the pan for 5-10 minutes.

6. In a microwave-safe bowl, combine the mashed blueberries, honey, and water. Microwave for 15-20 seconds, then mix until combined.

7. Spread the blueberry glaze over the top of the cornbread.

8. Let the cornbread come to room temperature before slicing and serving.

9. Enjoy!

Total Servings	12
Per Serving	
Calories	100
Added Sugar	5.9g
Fiber	1.2g
Fat	2.1g
Saturated Fat	1.2g
Protein	2.9g

Values are approximate and may vary based on ingredients used

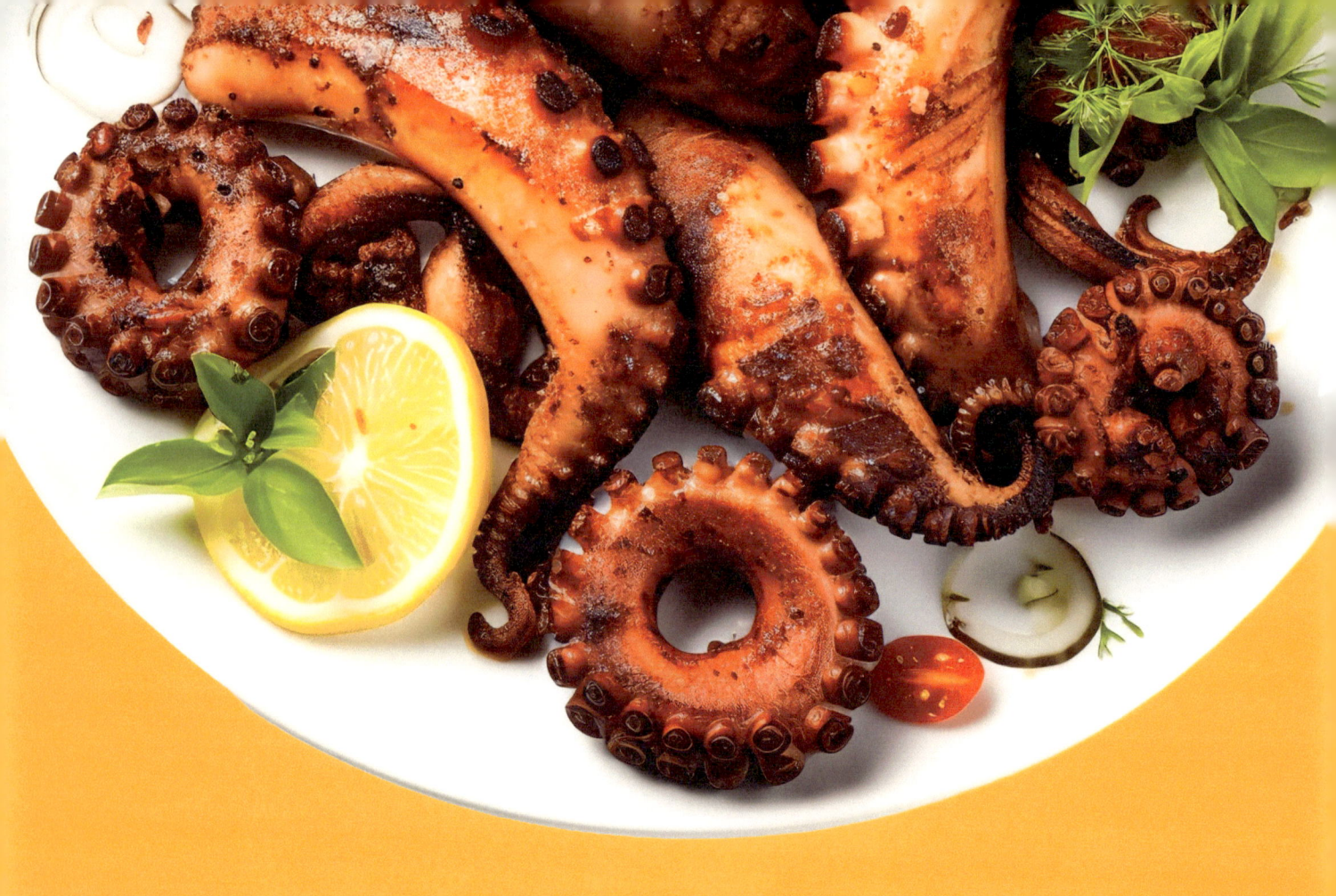

LEMON AND OREGANO OCTOPUS

LEMON AND OREGANO OCTOPUS

Try something new with this lemon and oregano octopus. Tender, flavorful, and perfect for a special meal.

INGREDIENTS

1 pound whole octopus

1 teaspoon dried oregano

1 lemon (½ sliced thin and the other half for juicing)

½ tablespoon olive oil

Salt to wash the octopus and to boil the octopus

METHOD

1. Remove the beak from the octopus.

2. In a large bowl, add plenty of water and a handful of salt. Add the octopus to the bowl and wash it thoroughly.

3. Bring a pot of water to a boil and add a pinch of salt.

4. Once boiling, hold the octopus by the area where the beak was removed and dip it in and out of the boiling water until the tentacles start to curl up. Once they start to curl, drop the octopus into the water, reduce heat to low, and cook for 30 minutes or until a knife can penetrate the tentacle without much resistance.

5. Remove the octopus from the water and cut it up as desired. I like to separate the tentacles and cut up the body.

6. Heat a pan until hot, then add the olive oil. Add the octopus to the pan, searing it for 2-3 minutes. Flip everything and juice ½ of a lemon into the pan. Mix everything around, then add the oregano and lemon slices. Cook for 1 more minute, stirring everything thoroughly.

7. Plate and enjoy!

Total Servings	2
Per Serving	
Calories	116
Added Sugar	0g
Fiber	1.2g
Fat	4.8g
Saturated Fat	0.5g
Protein	12.9g

Values are approximate and may vary based on ingredients used

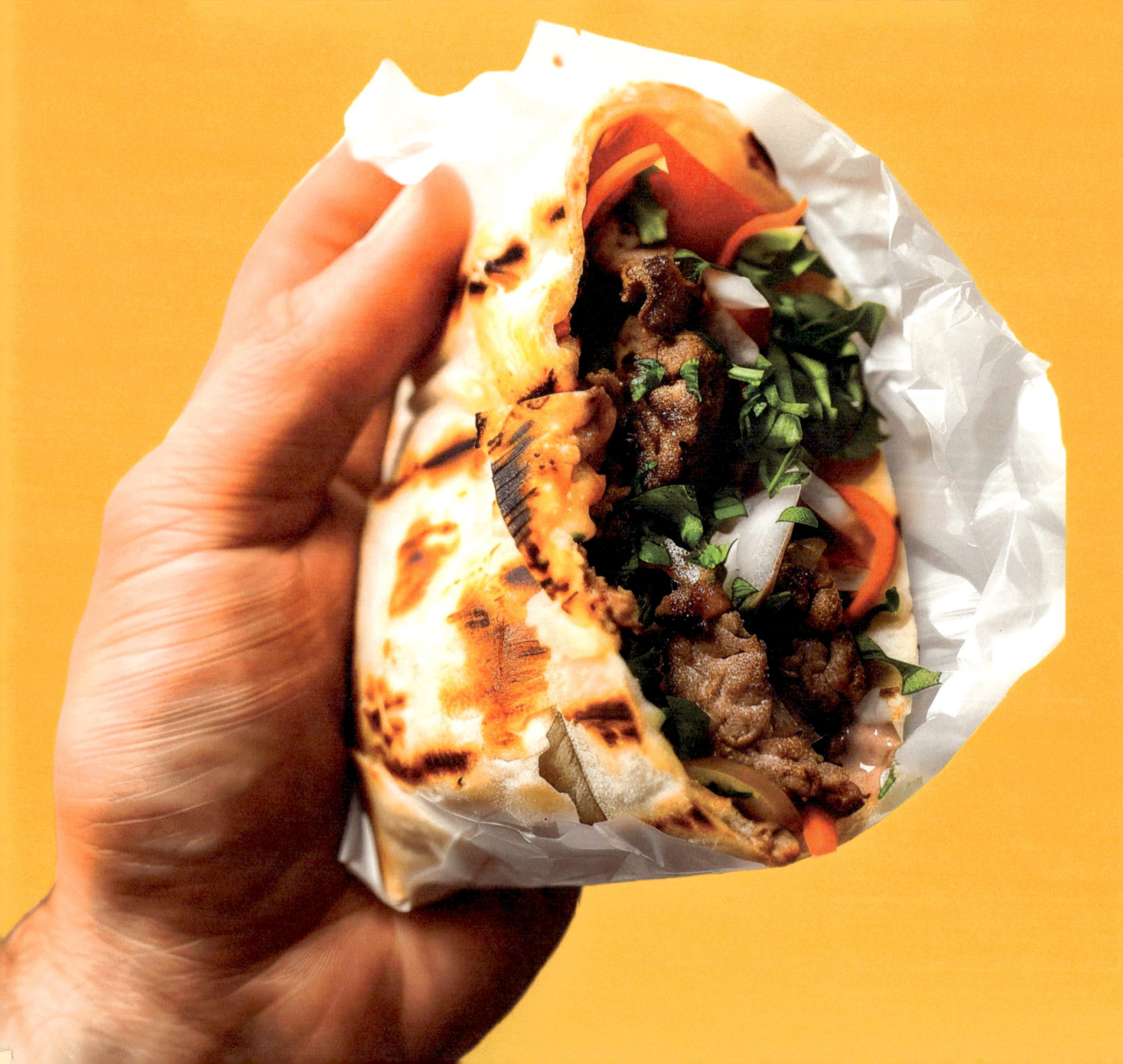

CHICKEN KEBAB WRAP

CHICKEN KEBAB WRAP

Juicy, flavorful chicken kebab wraps are perfect for a quick, tasty meal. So good!

INGREDIENTS

1 pound ground chicken

¼ cup finely chopped fresh parsley (half for kebab and half for topping)

¼ cup finely diced yellow onion

6 garlic cloves, mashed into a paste (or 1 tablespoon garlic paste)

½ yellow onion, grated

1 tablespoon hot pepper paste

¼ teaspoon cumin

¼ teaspoon allspice

¼ teaspoon coriander

¼ teaspoon turmeric

¼ teaspoon dried oregano

¼ teaspoon smoked paprika

½ cup non-fat yogurt

2 tablespoons tahini

Salt and pepper to taste

6 whole-wheat flatbreads

6 pickle wedges, sliced lengthwise

1 large tomato, sliced

METHOD

1. In a bowl, combine the diced yellow onion and half of the chopped parsley. Set aside.

2. In a separate bowl, combine the yogurt and tahini. Season with salt and pepper, then set aside.

3. Squeeze out all the liquid from the grated onion using a cheesecloth. Add the onion to a cutting board along with the remaining chopped parsley. Chop the mixture even finer.

4. In a large bowl, combine the finely chopped onion and parsley mixture with the hot pepper paste, cumin, allspice, coriander, turmeric, dried oregano, smoked paprika, and ground chicken. Mix well.

5. Portion out the mixture into 6 equal thick sausage-shaped pieces, about 4-5 inches long.

6. Heat a pan over medium-high heat and add olive oil. Once hot, add two kebab pieces and cook for 3 minutes on each side, ensuring all sides are cooked until the internal temperature reaches 165°F. Repeat for all pieces.

7. To assemble the wrap, spread some of the yogurt-tahini sauce on a piece of flatbread. Add some of the parsley and onion mixture, tomato slices, and pickles. Place 2 kebab pieces on top.

8. Wrap it up tightly and enjoy!

Total Servings	6
Per Serving	
Calories	253.2
Added Sugar	0g
Fiber	3.9g
Fat	10.5g
Saturated Fat	2.2g
Protein	17.4g

Values are approximate and may vary based on ingredients used

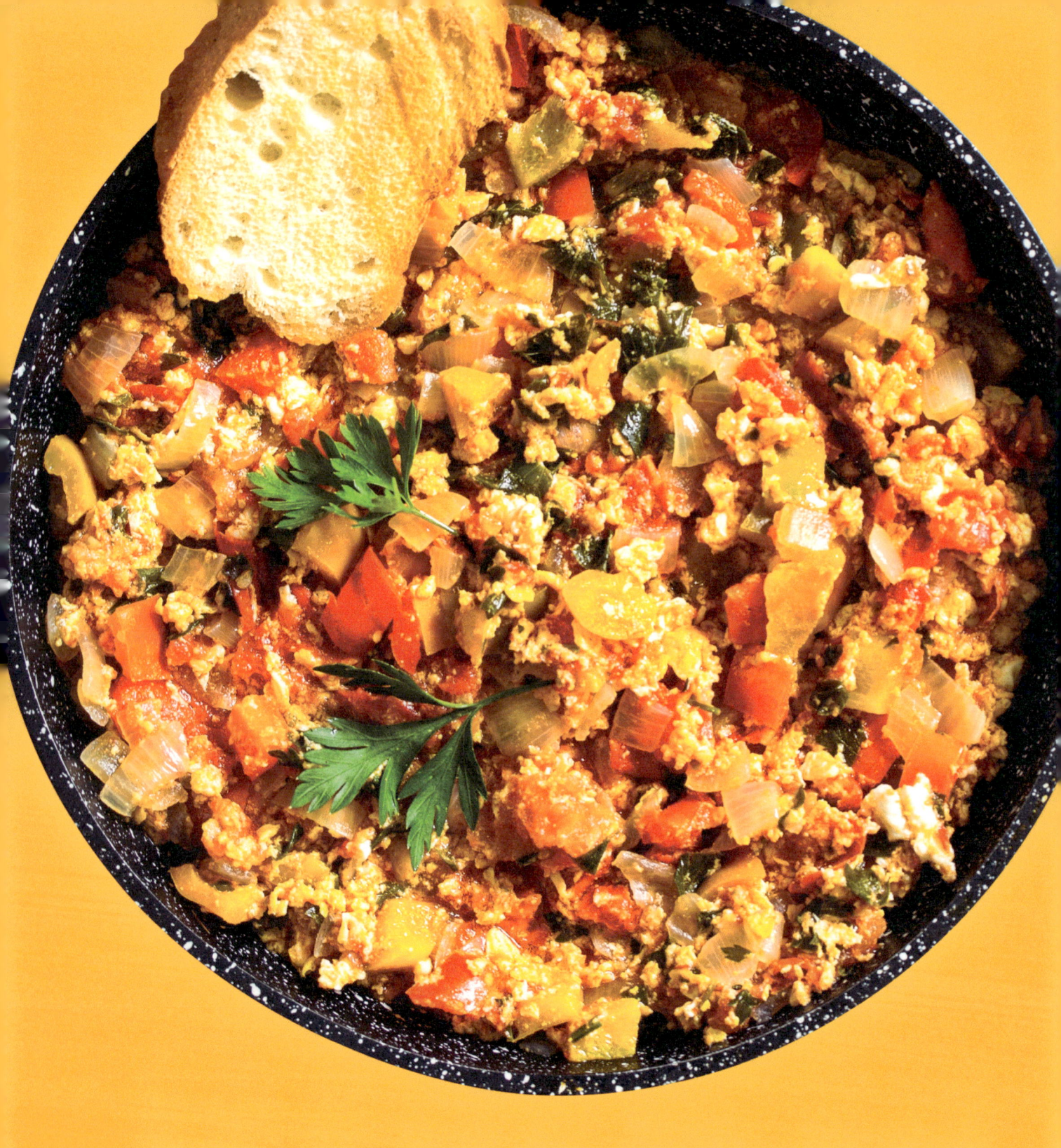

MENEMEN

MENEMEN

Start your day with this delicious, savory menemen. A Turkish breakfast dish that's packed with flavor.

INGREDIENTS

4 large tomatoes or 1 pound tomatoes, diced

1 red bell pepper, diced

3 large eggs

1 Calabrian chili, deseeded, stem removed, and sliced

1 tablespoon olive oil

Salt and pepper to taste

METHOD

1. Heat olive oil in a pan over medium heat. Add the diced red bell pepper and sliced Calabrian chili. Sauté for 5-6 minutes, or until soft.

2. Add the diced tomatoes to the pan and cook for 7 minutes, or until they start releasing their juices.

3. While the tomatoes are cooking, whisk the eggs in a bowl.

4. Once the tomatoes start releasing their juices, add the whisked eggs to the pan. Stir rapidly until the eggs are just set.

5. Season with salt and pepper to taste.

6. Enjoy!

Total Servings	2
Per Serving	
Calories	255.5
Added Sugar	0g
Fiber	6.7g
Fat	15.3g
Saturated Fat	3.6g
Protein	13g

Values are approximate and may vary based on ingredients used

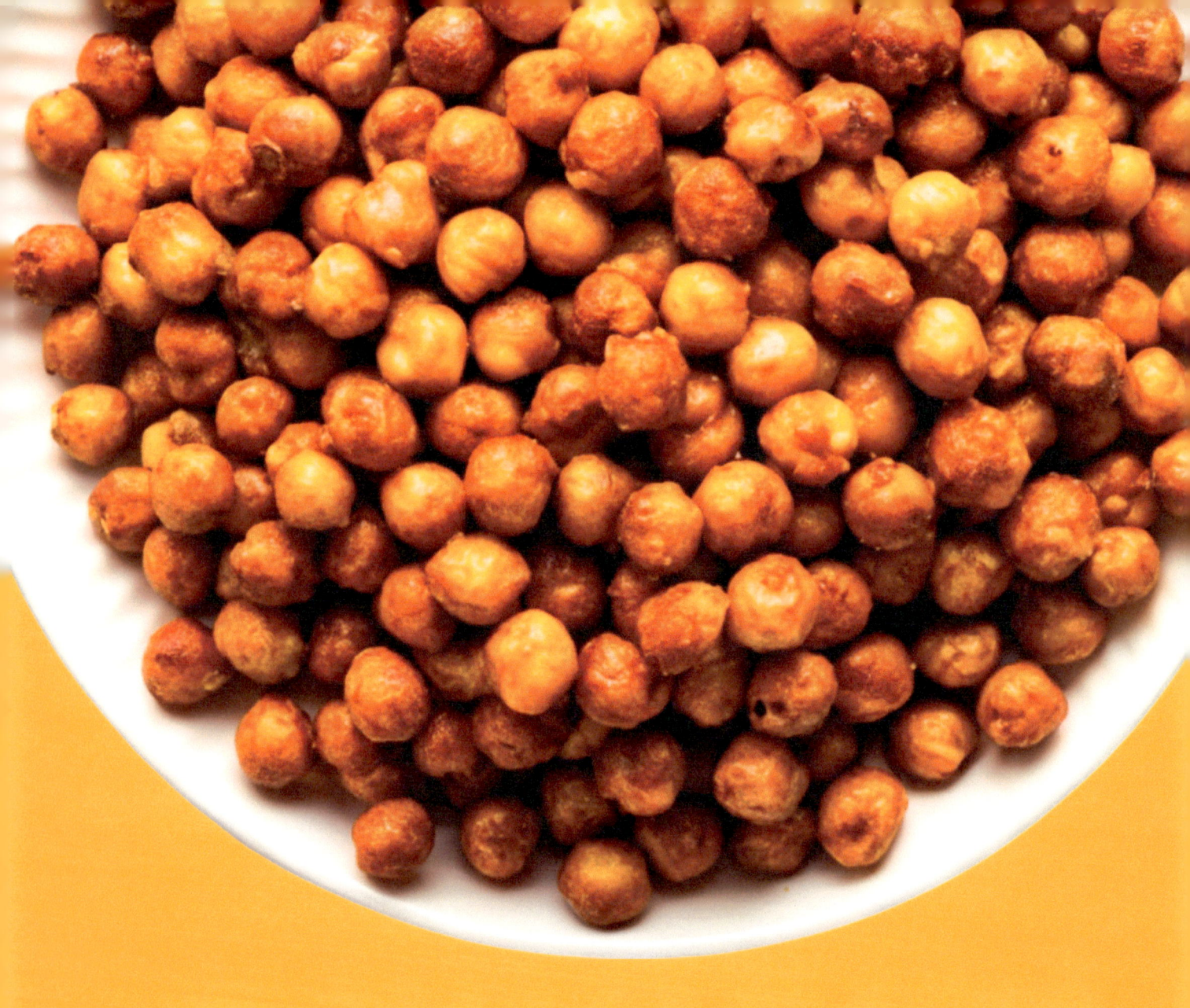

CRUNCHY CHICKPEAS

CRUNCHY CHICKPEA SNACK

These crunchy chickpeas are a great savory snack—crispy, flavorful, and totally addictive!

INGREDIENTS

15 oz can of chickpeas

2.5 tablespoons avocado oil

½ teaspoon smoked paprika

¼ teaspoon garlic powder

¼ teaspoon onion powder

Salt and pepper to taste

METHOD

1. Preheat the oven to 425°F. Line a baking sheet with parchment paper. Drain and rinse the chickpeas, then pat them dry with towels.

2. In a large skillet, heat the avocado oil over medium-high heat. Add the chickpeas and cook for 5 to 8 minutes, stirring occasionally until they are blistered and slightly charred. Drain any remaining oil.

3. Transfer the chickpeas to the prepared baking sheet. Bake for 17 to 20 minutes, or until they are light golden brown and crispy.

4. Remove from the oven and sprinkle the smoked paprika, garlic powder, onion powder, salt, and pepper over the chickpeas. Toss them in the spices.

5. Return the chickpeas to the oven for an additional 5 minutes.

6. Cool slightly before serving.

7. Enjoy!

Total Servings	4
Per Serving	
Calories	138
Added Sugar	0g
Fiber	2.7g
Fat	9.6g
Saturated Fat	1.2g
Protein	3.6g

Values are approximate and may vary based on ingredients used

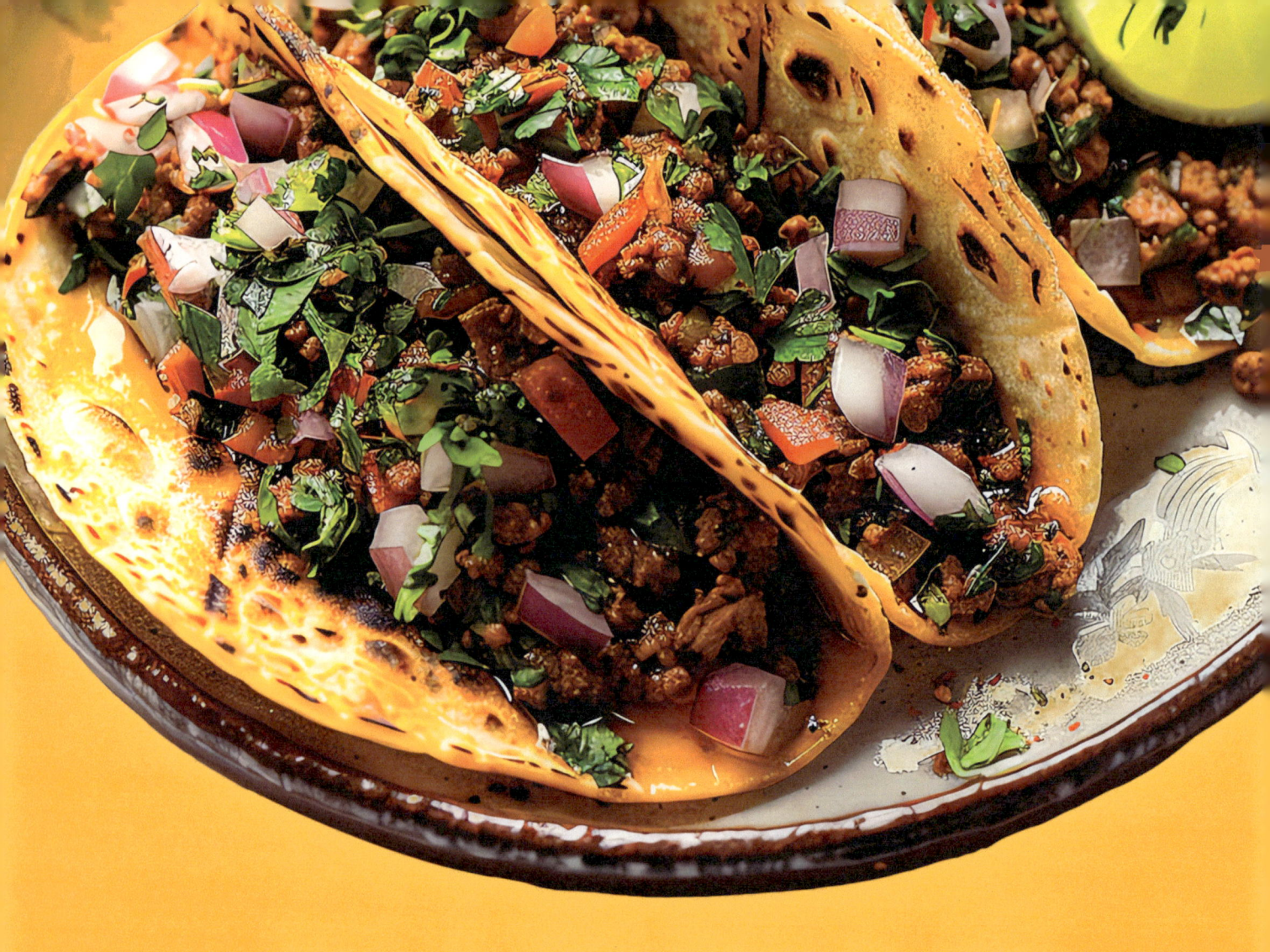

BIRRIA TACOS

BIRRIA TACOS

These Birria Tacos are packed with tender beef and melty cheese, perfect for dipping in a flavorful broth. Your taco nights will never be the same!

INGREDIENTS

2 lb beef shank

1 tablespoon tomato paste

1 yellow onion, chopped

7 cloves garlic

2 quarts beef stock

1 bay leaf

1 teaspoon (4g) cumin seeds

2 teaspoons (8g) black peppercorns

2 teaspoons (8g) oregano

1 cinnamon stick

4 ancho chilies

4 guajillo chilies

2 chili de árbol

Salt to taste

16 low-carb corn tortillas, for serving

2 cups (240g) shredded low moisture part skim mozzarella cheese

Total Servings	8
Per Serving	
Calories	448
Carbohydrates	22g
Fiber	7g
Fat	12g
Saturated Fat	4g
Protein	42g

Values are approximate and may vary based on ingredients used

METHOD

1. Debone and then cut the meat into 2-inch cubes. Pat the meat dry with a paper towel and season with salt and pepper.

2. Spray a large pot with cooking spray and set over medium-high heat. In batches, sear the beef until browned on all sides. Remove the beef from the pot and reserve. Reduce heat to medium.

3. Add tomato paste to the pot and stir constantly until lightly caramelized, around 30 seconds. Add chopped onion and garlic, sauté for 30 seconds.

4. Add beef stock and increase heat to medium-high to bring to a boil. Reduce heat to low, add the reserved beef back into the pot, and add one bay leaf.

5. Place cumin seeds, black peppercorns, oregano, and one cinnamon stick in a cheesecloth, wrap it up, and tie with butcher's twine. Drop the spice bundle into the pot.

6. Add ancho chilies, guajillo chilies, chili de árbol, and a generous pinch of salt to the pot. Cover and let simmer for 4-5 hours, or until the beef is extremely tender.

7. Carefully remove the chilies and place them in a blender along with 2 cups of braising liquid. Remove and discard the garlic, onion, and bay leaf. Blend the chilies on high and pour the mixture back into the pot.

8. Remove the beef from the pot and place it in a large mixing bowl. Shred by hand until very fine and season with salt to taste. Add a spoonful of broth to the beef and mix.

9. To make tacos, heat a large heavy-bottomed pan over medium heat. Grease generously with cooking spray. Once hot, dunk a corn tortilla in the broth, then place it on the hot pan.

10. Add mozzarella cheese on one side of the tortilla, followed by beef. Fold the tortilla over to form a mini quesadilla. Cook for 1-2 minutes, flip, and cook for another 1-2 minutes until crispy and brown.

11. Serve with lime wedges and a ramekin of broth on the side for dipping.

12. Enjoy!

Made in the USA
Columbia, SC
16 December 2024